External Ventricular and Lumbar Drains

External Ventricular and Lumbar Drains

INDICATIONS, PROCEDURES, AND PATIENT CARE

REDI RAHMANI, MD
Department of Neurosurgery
University of Rochester
Rochester, New York

MICHAEL T. LAWTON, MD
Department of Neurosurgery
Barrow Neurological Institute
St. Joseph's Hospital and Medical Center
Phoenix, Arizona

G. EDWARD VATES, MD, PhD
Department of Neurosurgery
University of Rochester
Rochester, New York

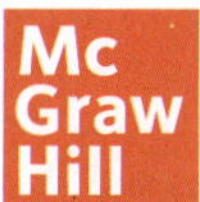

New York Chicago San Francisco Athens London Madrid Mexico City
Milan New Delhi Singapore Sydney Toronto

External Ventricular and Lumbar Drains: Indications, Procedures, and Patient Care

Copyright © 2024 by McGraw Hill LLC. All rights reserved. Printed in China. Except as permitted under the United States Copyright Act of 1976, no part of this publication may be reproduced or distributed in any form or by any means, or stored in a data base or retrieval system, without the prior written permission of the publisher.

1 2 3 4 5 6 7 8 9   DSS   28 27 26 25 24 23

ISBN 978-1-264-26829-0
MHID 1-264-26829-7

This book was set in Minion Pro by MPS Limited.
The editors were Timothy Y. Hiscock and Peter J. Boyle.
The production supervisor was Richard Ruzycka.
Project management was provided by Poonam Bisht, MPS Limited.
Cover art by Aaron Cole, MS

Barrow Neurological Institute holds the copyright to all diagnostic images, photographs, intraoperative videos, animations, and art (including the cover art) used in this work and the accompanying digital content, unless otherwise stated. Used with permission from Barrow Neurological Institute, Phoenix, Arizona.

The authors have no personal, financial, or institutional interest in any of the drugs, materials, or devices described in this book.

Library of Congress Control Number: 2023938249

McGraw Hill books are available at special quantity discounts to use as premiums and sales promotions or for use in corporate training programs. To contact a representative, please visit the Contact Us pages at www.mhprofessional.com.

To my parents, who taught me that with hard work and honesty, any goal is achievable.

—Redi Rahmani, MD

To all my residents—past, present, and future—who help me manage this underappreciated aspect of neurosurgical care.

—Michael T. Lawton, MD

To the neurosurgery residents—past, present, and future—at the University of Rochester.

—G. Edward Vates, MD, PhD

CONTENTS

Cerebral spinal fluid (CSF) diversion via external ventricular drain (EVD) or lumbar drain (LD) placement is frequently the first-line neurosurgical intervention for patients with acute brain injuries. Drain placement allows for emergent relief of brain compression and intracranial hypertension, at times stabilizing a patient for the operating room or even preventing the need for further neurosurgical intervention. These procedures provide the benefits of CSF drainage, intracranial pressure monitoring, and intrathecal medication administration. With proper insertion and management, these drains can remain in place for up to 21 days with minimal infection risk.

The often life-saving procedure of CSF drain placement is the most visible neurosurgical procedure to other medical services when collaboratively managing patients with brain injuries. Many such patients are admitted to the intensive care unit for close monitoring and management. Intensivists and the intensive care team must have expert knowledge of the placement techniques, potential risks, troubleshooting tactics, and ongoing management of CSF drains to prevent infection, provide effective communication with the neurosurgical team, and yield the best possible outcomes for the patients. EVD and LD weaning and clamping trials can lead to neurologic deterioration if the patient is not appropriately monitored. Therefore, a collaborative approach to EVD or LD management is most beneficial.

Drain placement is commonly the first neurosurgical procedure performed by neurosurgery trainees, and they will likely place well over 100 drains throughout a busy neurosurgery residency. These procedures, done at the bedside of an actively deteriorating patient, are often associated with high stress for the clinician. Dr. Rahmani and his notable colleagues adeptly describe the thrill and terror associated with such a procedure in the Introduction.

This book is a superlative handbook that details the intricacies of CSF drainage. Perched at the intersection of neurosurgery and neurocritical care, *External Ventricular and Lumbar Drains: Indications, Procedures, and Patient Care* guides all clinicians who interact with CSF drainage devices to best practices. We applaud the authors for their dedication to this essential yet often-overlooked topic.

Debra E. Roberts, MD, PhD
Medical Director, Neurocritical Care
Fellowship Director, Neurocritical Care
University of Rochester Medical Center
Rochester, New York

Webster H. Pilcher, MD, PhD
Ernest and Thelma Del Monte Distinguished
Professor of Neuromedicine
Chair, Department of Neurosurgery
University of Rochester Medical Center
Rochester, New York

Learning to place an external ventricular drain (EVD) has long been considered a rite of passage for those training to become neurosurgeons. Although I have placed many EVDs in my career, I can still recall placing my first one as an intern. Before me in the emergency department lay a moribund patient with a large ventricular hemorrhage from a ruptured intracranial aneurysm. My nervousness translated to ice-cold fingers that felt unable to perform the procedure correctly and made me think I was not moving fast enough. My ears rang with the hum of monitors, alarms, the ventilator, and the medical staff around me talking. My mind raced as I reviewed the steps of the procedure and the equipment checklist.

At this point, a crowd of onlookers had gathered in the emergency department. Nursing students and battle-hardened critical care nurses alike had congregated to watch the neurosurgeon "save the patient's life." For many, this experience would be the closest that they would ever come to seeing what we do as neurosurgeons in such a dramatic fashion. With so many eyes upon me, I wondered if they realized that I felt like an imposter. This person who had been sent to save the patient had minimal experience and practically no idea of what he was doing. Could they not see my hesitation and my every blunder?

As I made the first cut, blood gushed from the scalp feeders. This incision, which I had been taught was more than sufficient for the entire procedure, seemed grossly inadequate because the pool of briskly flowing blood offered no glimpse of the underlying bone. Two gauze pads later and with no progress yet in controlling the bleeding, I felt the eyes of the onlookers burning into my forehead while a cold sweat enveloped me. Despite the bleeding, I decided to press forward with the drilling.

To this day, the push-pull routine of the drill feels unnatural. It requires all the strength in your hands, yet must be gentle enough at just the right moment so that you do not plunge into the underlying brain. The "release" of the drill as the inner cortex opened was my first small victory in what seemed to be an eternity since the procedure had started.

After the dura was opened and placement of the EVD began, the moment of truth arrived. For the first time in my life, I felt the parting of brain tissue at the tip of the drain. The resistance from the density of the white matter and the wall of the ventricle engendered self-doubt that I had completed an accurate trajectory. Was I just blindly wandering around in this patient's brain? But I summoned the fortitude to press forward, never more in tune with the pads of my fingers, until I felt the unmistakable "pop"—the ultimate victory. Blood-tinged cerebrospinal fluid began emanating from the end of the drain. Without a word, everyone watching understood that the procedure had been successful.

The EVD bedside procedure, like the placement of the lumbar drain (LD), is one of the most frequently performed procedures conducted by neurosurgeons and neurosurgery residents, often in life-saving circumstances. Having performed more than 100 of these procedures myself, I believe that placing these two types of drains is also the most common point of contact between neurosurgeons and the practitioners of other medical specialties. Many of the neurosurgeon's daily interactions with other members of the medical team involve troubleshooting and managing EVDs and LDs.

This book is intended to be the definitive manual for the placement and management of both types of drains. In its chapters, my coauthors and I enumerate the planning and procedure stages for each drain and then examine the problems that arise and how to troubleshoot them. Relevant examples from our training, experience, and background are provided to enhance the lessons we aim to teach.

Our goal is not to remove neurosurgeons from the equation and allow other members of the medical team to place and manage EVDs and LDs independently but instead to convey the rationale of their management. Therefore, this book is intended for more than junior neurosurgery residents who are just learning how to place these drains. It has also been written for emergency, critical care, interventional radiology, anesthesia, and neurology residents, fellows, advanced practice providers, and attendings, as well as for critical care nurses, transport medics, and medical students who may be assisting with patient care.

The three of us hope you will both enjoy and learn from this book. We welcome your feedback on how to improve its content in later editions.

Redi Rahmani, MD

We thank the staff of Neuroscience Publications at Barrow Neurological Institute for assistance with manuscript preparation, including Samantha Soto and Laura Repak for assistance with manuscript preparation and coordination, Aaron Cole and Cassie Todd for medical illustrations, and Paula Card Higginson and Lynda Orescanin for editorial assistance. We also thank Mary Ann Clifft (EditWrite, LLC) for editorial assistance and Aleta Pennington for proofreading. We are grateful to Jeanette S. McCorry, PA-C; Nathaniel R. Ellens, MD; Jessica Hasenauer, RN, BSN, CCRN; Catherine R. G. Jay, MD; Catherine A. Gargan, RN, BSN, CNRN, CCRN; Lauren M. Paganin, RN, BSN, CCRN; Andrew Tsavaris, CANPC-AG; Gurkirat S. Kohli, MD; Taylor J. Furst, MD; Derek D. George, MD; Clifton Houk, MD; Gabrielle C. Santangelo, MD; Catherine E. Wassef, MD; David A. Paul, MD; Thomas A. Pieters, MD; Visish M. Srinivasan, MD; Joshua S. Catapano, MD; Irakliy Abramov, MD, PhD; Lea Scherschinski, MD; Katherine Karahalios, MS; Mohamed A. Labib, MD, CM; and Stephen S. Susa, BA for their help drafting the content and obtaining the clinical images.

DISCLOSURES: The authors have no personal, financial, or institutional interest in any of the drugs, materials, or devices described in this book.

FINANCIAL SUPPORT: None

FRONT MATTER PERMISSION LINES: Cover art by Aaron Cole, MS. Barrow Neurological Institute holds the copyright to all diagnostic images, photographs, intraoperative videos, animations, and art (including the cover art) used in this work and the accompanying digital content, unless otherwise stated. Used with permission from Barrow Neurological Institute, Phoenix, Arizona.

External Ventricular and Lumbar Drains

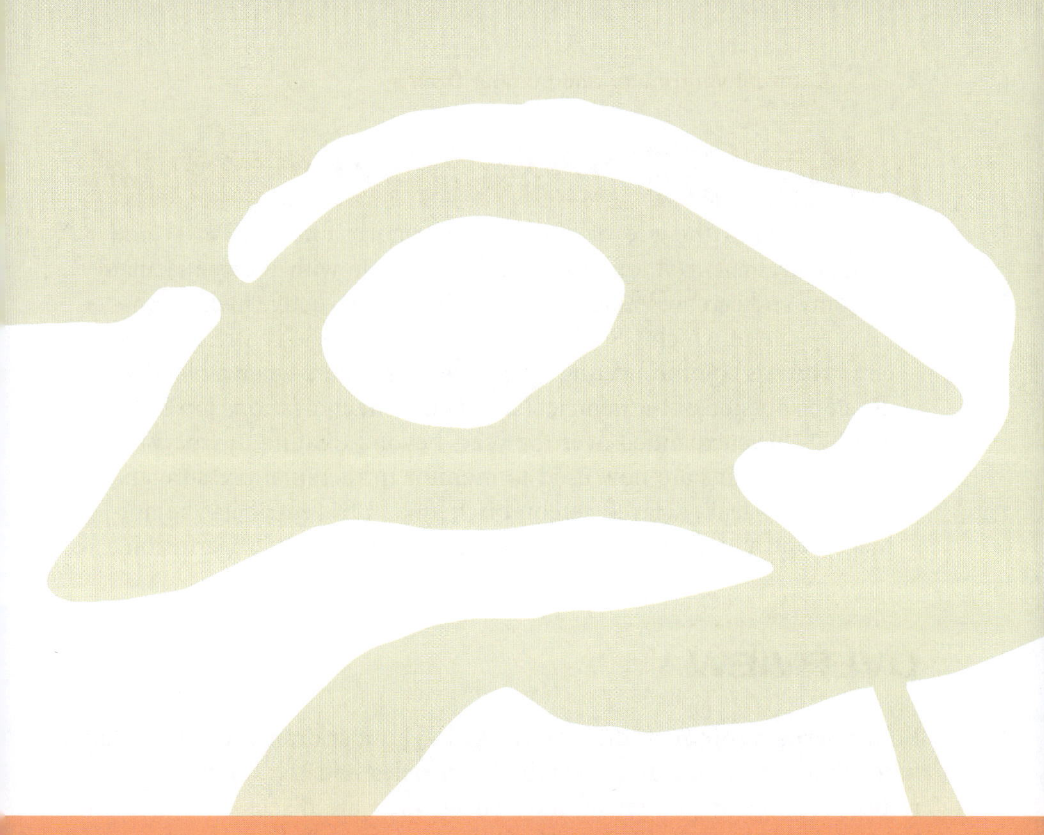

CHAPTER 1

Indications

CHAPTER SUMMARY

To understand the use of external ventricular drains (EVDs) and lumbar drains (LDs), one must be comfortable with the ventricular anatomy and cerebrospinal fluid (CSF) flow. Obstructive hydrocephalus is a state in which CSF flow is blocked within the ventricular system, whereas communicating hydrocephalus occurs when a blockage develops outside of the ventricular system. The indications for EVDs and LDs have expanded over the years beyond treating hydrocephalus. These drains are now used to monitor intracranial pressure and to treat CSF leak, delayed cerebral ischemia, intraventricular hemorrhage, central nervous system infection, and spinal cord reperfusion.

OVERVIEW

Both external ventricular drains (EVDs) and lumbar drains (LDs) are thin tubes that are placed in the cerebral ventricles and the lumbar cistern, respectively. Their placement and management are discussed in greater detail in later chapters. EVDs and LDs have historically been used to treat hydrocephalus. However, their roles have expanded for other purposes, including intracranial pressure (ICP) management, repair of cerebrospinal fluid (CSF) leak, and drug delivery.

CSF ANATOMY

The conceptualization of hydrocephalus will likely undergo a major restructuring within the next 50 years.[1] Increasing evidence shows that rather than the bulk fluid flow model, which has been prevailing for decades, a pulsation model may more accurately describe CSF dynamics. However, because the pulsation model has not yet been fully elucidated, we will refer to the classic thinking that is most often used in the medical literature. Hydrocephalus is a state involving the disruption of the normal pathway of CSF movement. The most clinically relevant way to conceptualize this disruption is to identify where it has occurred within that pathway. Establishing this mental blueprint can help answer many of the questions that arise about the different types of hydrocephalus and their management with drains. Thus, we must become intimately familiar with the anatomy of CSF movement.

One can imagine CSF flow as a lake system, similar to the rivers and gorges making up the Finger Lakes in upstate New York. CSF is produced predominantly in the specialized cells of the choroid plexus of the ventricles (although this source has become a topic of debate).[2] These slightly transparent beige tufts of choroidal epithelial cells are much like the many small streams and brooks that join to form a river (Fig. 1.1). For the most part, CSF flow is continuous, as is the case with tributaries. The first two rivers can be thought of as existing in the lateral ventricles. As CSF moves along the different parts of the lateral ventricle, the choroid plexus along the medial-inferior wall continues to add more CSF to these hypothetical rivers. The two rivers join at the beginning of the third ventricle as they pass through the foramen of Monro. Here, too, CSF moves downstream, and more small brooks join from the choroid plexus along the roof of the third ventricle. CSF continues into a much narrower segment called the sylvian aqueduct. The river then opens into the larger fourth ventricle, with small tributaries continuing to add to it from the choroid plexus along the roof of the ventricle formed by the cerebellum. Finally, the river reaches its delta as it empties into the lake. The delta consists of the lateral foramen of Luschka and the more medially occurring foramen of Magendie. The lake is large, and spans from the very bottom of the lumbar cistern in the lower back to the top of the brain to include all the named basilar cisterns (Fig. 1.2). Just as some lakes have one or more dams to control the water level, our CSF lake system has a dam as well, which is represented by arachnoid granulations in the dural sinuses (Fig. 1.3). Recent investigations have questioned the unidirectional flow of CSF; thus, we can think of absorption as occurring predominantly along the banks of the streams, rivers, and lakes and as being less dependent on the driving pressure of the fluid.[3,4] Our bodies produce 0.3 to 0.4 mL of CSF per minute, for a total production of 430 to 580 mL per day. The total volume of this entire "lake system" is approximately 160 mL, with 25 mL located within the ventricles. Therefore, the entire volume of the system is turned over every 6 to 9 hours.[4] The keys to understanding hydrocephalus in the classic model are to determine where the dam is located and how high its wall is.

OBSTRUCTIVE HYDROCEPHALUS

In obstructive hydrocephalus, the dam can be located anywhere before our theoretical river system empties into the lake. For the condition to be considered obstructive, the dam must completely prevent the movement of the river. As in the natural world when a dam is placed, a once-thin river

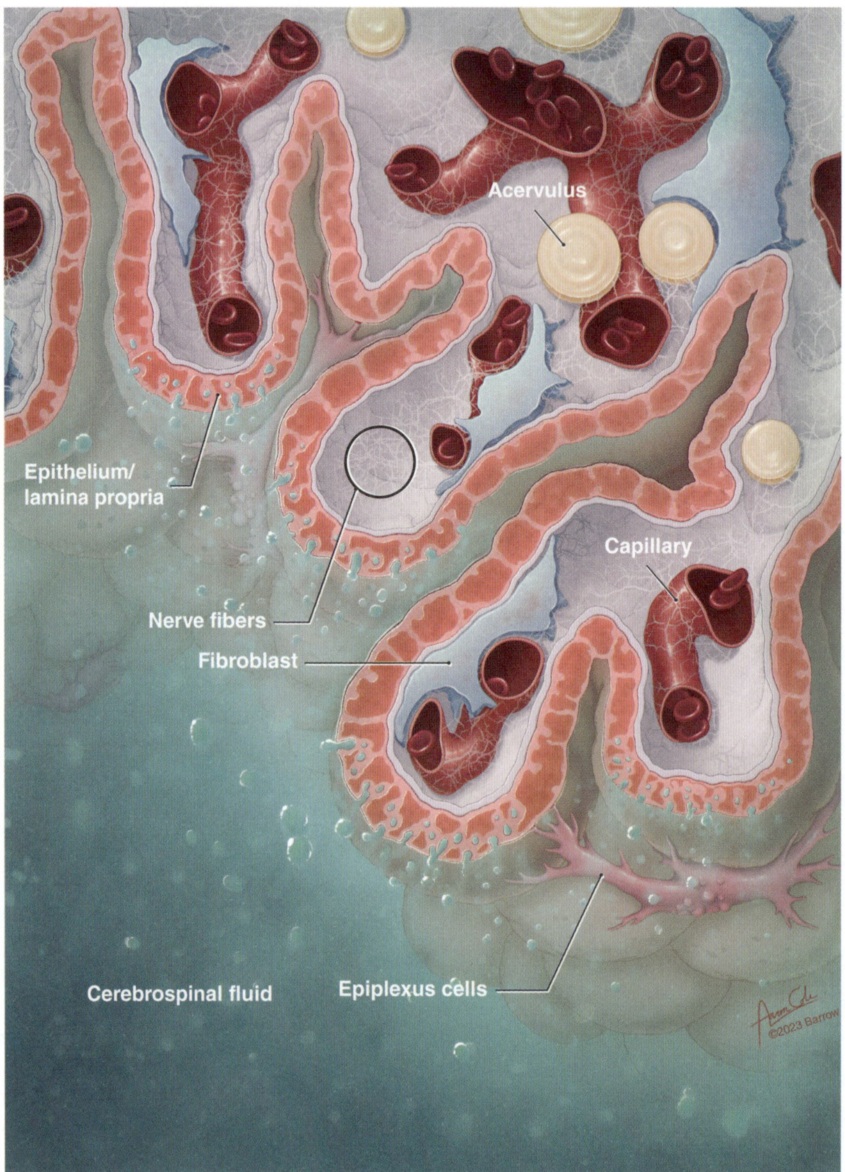

FIGURE 1.1. Choroidal epithelial cells producing cerebrospinal fluid (CSF). Artist's rendition of CSF production through choroid cells merging to form larger and larger streams of CSF emptying into the ventricles.

begins to overflow its banks, forming a body of water many times larger than the original. When this overflow occurs in the ventricular system, it causes CSF to overpower its walls and occupy more space than it would in its normal state.

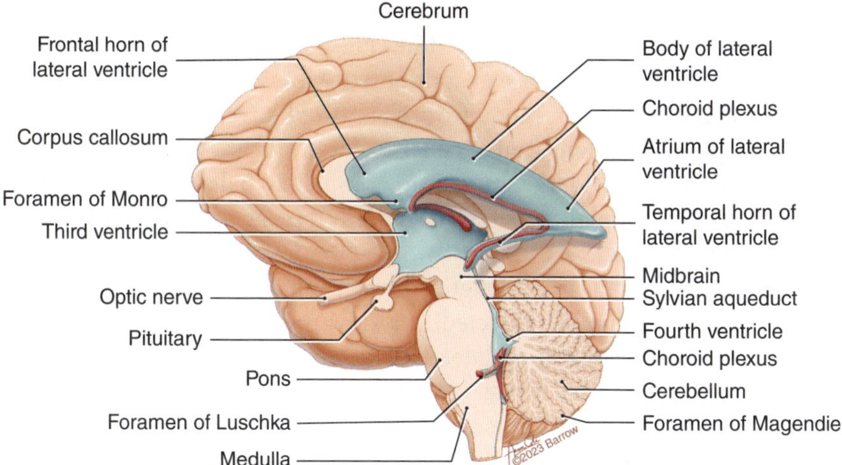

FIGURE 1.2. Anatomy of the ventricular system. Illustration of the human ventricular system showing the two lateral ventricles meeting at the third ventricle through the foramen of Monro. The third ventricle connects with the fourth ventricle through the sylvian aqueduct. From there, it communicates with the spinal and basilar cisterns through the foramina of Luschka and Magendie.

It is this increase in occupied space that leads to the clinical sequelae observed in the hydrocephalic patient. The intracranial space, which is enclosed completely by bone, has a finite volume. When one part of the system enlarges, it exerts pressure on the others, compressing them to accommodate the change. If the obstruction occurs in either of the lateral ventricles, then only that ventricle will enlarge. If it occurs only at the opening of the foramen of Monro, then both lateral ventricles will enlarge.

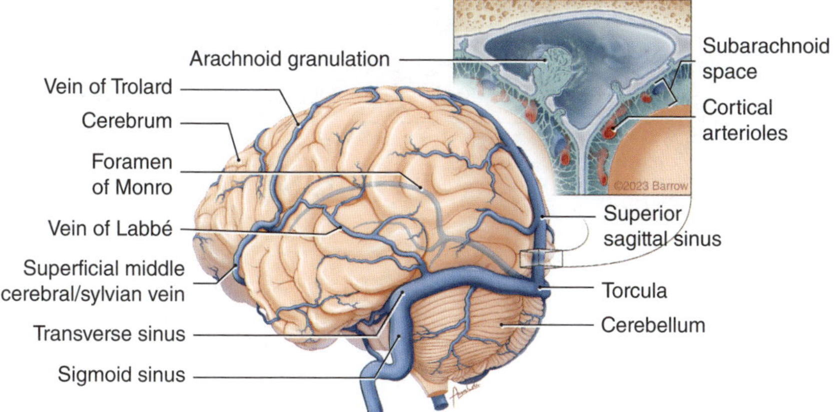

FIGURE 1.3. Anatomy of dural sinuses. Illustration of the dural sinuses, the major draining veins of the skull, which contain ports (*inset*) called *arachnoid granulations* that allow cerebrospinal fluid to drain into the venous system.

This logic can be followed all the way to the delta of our river formed by the foramina of Luschka and Magendie (Fig. 1.4).

Clinically, the dam can be represented by any number of entities. It may consist of ventricular blood from a ruptured intracranial aneurysm or a vascular malformation. It may consist of a tumor mass or an infectious source that has grown large enough to completely halt CSF flow. Scarred tissue from development, previous trauma, and surgery can also form walls impenetrable to CSF.

Equally important in obstructive hydrocephalus is the speed at which it develops. The brain, if subjected to a slow increase in pressure, will go to great lengths to accommodate. This accommodation produces striking anatomical rearrangements but minimal clinical effects. In contrast, a quick change in pressure or compression usually manifests with equally swift neurologic changes.

For patients in whom hydrocephalus develops quickly, the role of EVDs is most salient. An EVD must be placed upstream of the blockage to give an alternative route for CSF egress. This placement acts to lower the pressure in the blocked part of the ventricular system. In the classic model of obstructive hydrocephalus, an LD is not indicated. Using an LD is equivalent to draining our lake rather than the river above the dam, so it has no effect on reducing the fluid level above the blockage. Placing an

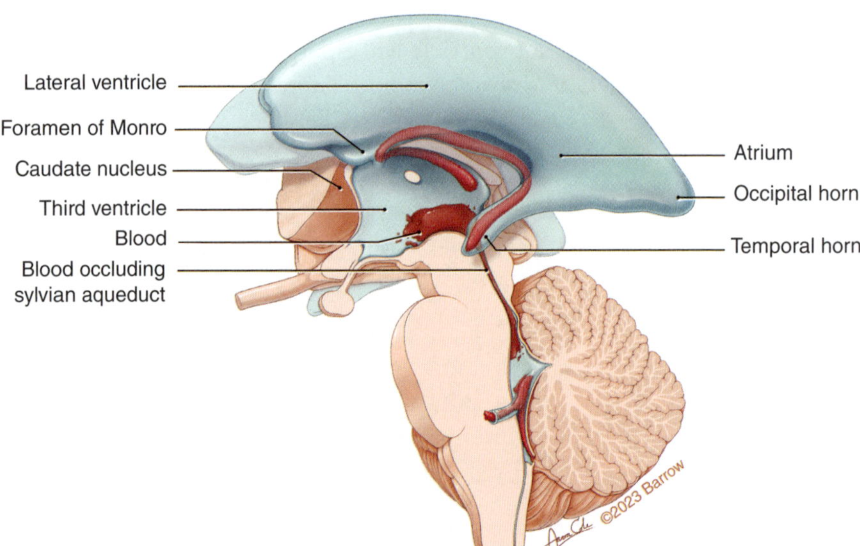

FIGURE 1.4. Occlusion of the sylvian aqueduct and enlargement of the ventricles. An illustrative obstruction of the aqueduct shows how a build-up of cerebrospinal fluid in the third ventricle and the lateral ventricles causes them to enlarge and exert increased pressure on the surrounding brain.

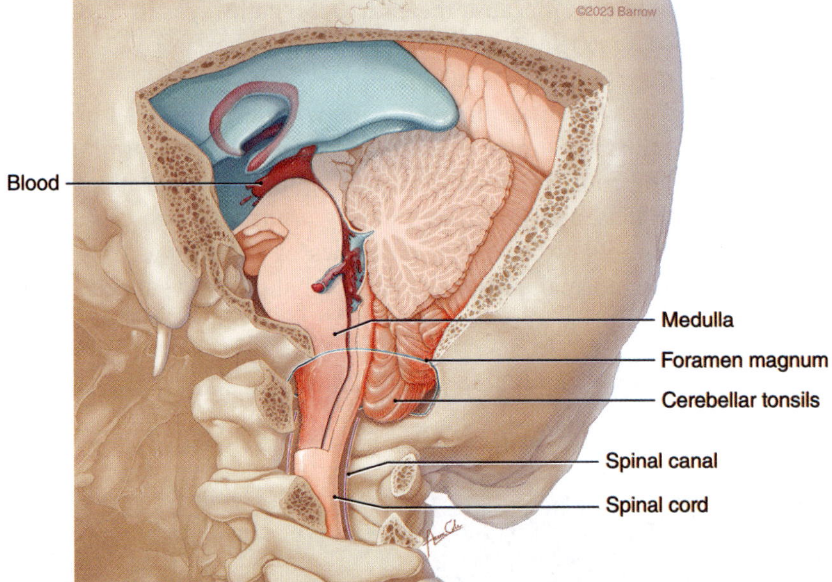

FIGURE 1.5. Brainstem herniation. When intracranial pressure exceeds the ability of the brain to compensate with deformation, part of the brain migrates through the foramen magnum in a process known as *tonsillar herniation* or *downward herniation*. This illustration demonstrates the condition, which has also been described in cases of overdrainage through a lumbar drain, with the brain being vacuumed down rather than being pushed down.

LD in a patient with obstructive hydrocephalus also poses the additional risk of herniation. In this exceptionally rare complication, a high-pressure gradient emanates from inside the cranial vault to the spinal canal. This pressure gradient is worsened by draining the CSF beyond the obstruction, such that eventually it overcomes the resistance of the brain to movement and is thus forced outside the skull into the spinal canal in a process known as *brain herniation* (Fig. 1.5).

COMMUNICATING HYDROCEPHALUS

In communicating hydrocephalus, the blockage occurs at the periphery of our large CSF lake, before it drains into the rivers (represented by the dural venous system of the brain). As mentioned previously, these draining rivers are represented anatomically by the arachnoid granulations. When the rivers are cluttered with debris, it causes the water level of the entire lake to rise, as well as the water level of the contributing brooks and streams. The types of debris include blood, protein products, and infectious organisms. Therefore, the solution is to circumvent the blockage along the arachnoid granulations. Because the entire CSF pathway is in "communication" from the ventricles to the basilar cistern, either an EVD or an LD will suffice in diverting CSF.

Communicating hydrocephalus has many different clinical presentations. It can occur after tumor resection, hemorrhage, or central nervous system (CNS) infection, with the theory being that tumor proteins, blood breakdown products, and postinflammatory products act to clog or dam the arachnoid granulations. Other examples of communicating hydrocephalus include normal pressure hydrocephalus, slit ventricle hydrocephalus, and hydrocephalus secondary to dural venous sinus stenosis or occlusion (Fig. 1.6).

An important distinction must be reinforced here. Previously, we defined obstructive hydrocephalus as a complete blockage in any part of

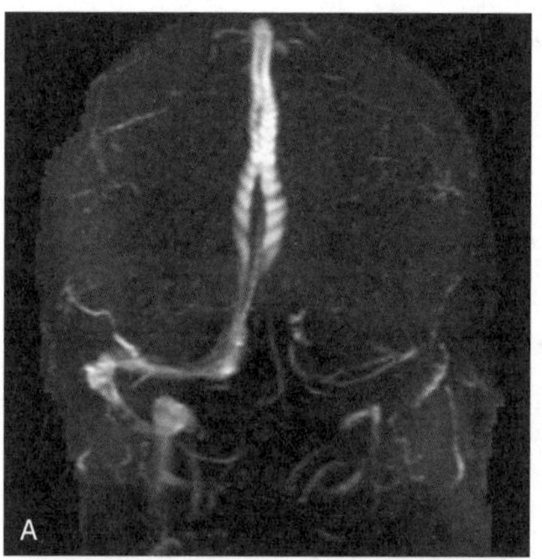

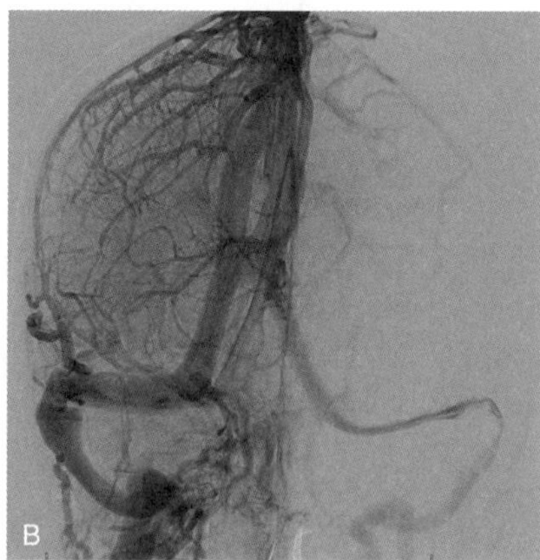

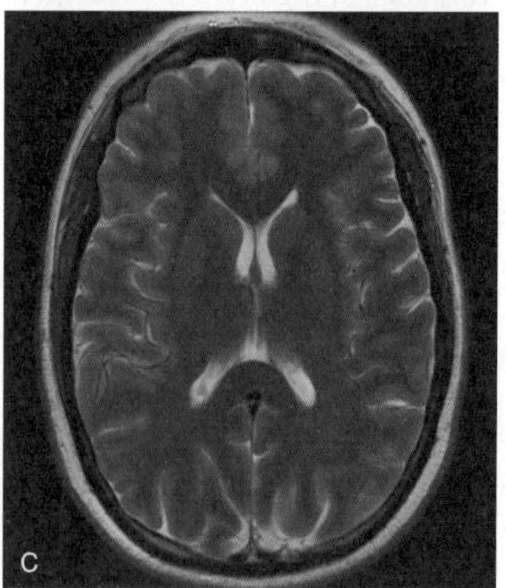

FIGURE 1.6. Communicating hydrocephalus. **A.** Magnetic resonance venogram (anteroposterior view) showing long-segment occlusion of the left transverse and sigmoid sinuses. This occlusion can be thought of as the damming of the lake, which causes water levels (ie, intracranial pressure) to rise in all locations. **B.** Digital subtraction catheter angiogram (anteroposterior view) showing the long-segment stenotic left transverse sigmoid sinus. **C.** In this case, the counterintuitive slit ventricle hydrocephalus has developed in the patient, as shown in the axial magnetic resonance image.

the system upstream from the large CSF lake. Even if this dam does not cause complete obstruction or the cessation of flow, it can cause relative obstruction, and the system can still be thought of as communicating. This distinction is important because it determines which drain is most appropriate and safest for the individual patient. Ultimately, if there is a question about the degree of obstruction, the EVD theoretically prevents the risk of herniation. However, even with a relatively blocked pathway such as the third or fourth ventricle, an LD can provide a safe treatment, and the amount of drainage chosen by the clinician can effectively lower ICP.[5]

ICP MONITORING

ICP is the pressure experienced by structures within the cranial vault. In most cases of hydrocephalus, either obstructive or communicating, ICP is elevated above normal. The now-famous Monro-Kellie doctrine, as summarized in 1926 by Cushing,[6] states that in an intact cranial vault, the total volume is fixed and is represented by the sum of the volumes of brain, CSF, and blood. Therefore, an increase in any one component necessitates a decrease in the other two components. The role of both the EVD and the LD is to facilitate the removal of CSF and allow this elevated ICP to normalize. However, these drain types not only divert CSF, they also directly measure the ICP.

This measurement is accomplished through a pressure transducer. CSF from the ventricles or the lumbar cistern travels through the tube of the drain into the pressure transducer chamber. This chamber consists of a thin membrane (usually made of silicone) that is part of an electrical circuit. On one side of the membrane is CSF and on the other is air. The air channel is zeroed (ie, made equivalent) to atmospheric pressure. A higher pressure in the CSF will bend this membrane down toward the channel with air, which changes the resistance in the circuit and the measured change is converted to a value (usually measured in mm Hg or cm H_2O).

Pressure measurements for both drains work on the principle of hydrostatic pressure:

$$p = \rho g h$$

where p = pressure in a fluid (N/m^2, Pa); ρ = density of the fluid (kg/m^3); g = acceleration of gravity (9.81 m/s^2); and h = height of fluid column.

This principle works only if the fluid column remains in continuity. In the case of ICP monitoring, the fluid column refers to the entirety of the

CSF from the point of interest to the pressure transducer. The density of CSF is assumed to be consistent throughout the two points. Therefore, the only factor that changes is h, the height of the fluid column. The height of the fluid column depends only on the difference in vertical distance from the point of interest to the transducer. The difference in vertical distance is important because the entrance points are different between the two types of drains, but the pressure will be equivalent as long as the height between the point of interest and the pressure transducer is the same. This principle was proved in 43 patients with intracranial hemorrhage who had nearly equivalent values at 0° and 30° positions, with and without vein compression (Fig. 1.7).[7]

Important consideration must once again be given to obstructive hydrocephalus and communicating hydrocephalus. As discussed previously, for fluid pressure transduction to be accurate, the fluid column must remain in continuity between the point of interest and the point measuring pressure. Therefore, in obstructive hydrocephalus, a catheter in the lumbar cistern will have a fluid column in discontinuity with the intracranial space, resulting in values that may not be accurate. Likewise, debris within the catheter or tube can create discontinuity in the fluid column, resulting in inaccurate values.

OTHER INDICATIONS

CSF Leak

The indications for both EVDs and LDs have increased over the past two decades. The classic indication for an LD remains the management of CSF leak. In a randomized controlled trial of patients undergoing intradural endoscopic skull base surgery, the postoperative use of an LD was found to significantly reduce the rate of CSF leak ($p = 0.02$).[8] In another randomized controlled trial, patients with traumatic CSF rhinorrhea who underwent LD drainage had a significantly reduced duration of rhinorrhea ($p = 0.001$).[9] Prophylactic antibiotics are not recommended for patients with basilar skull fractures and CSF leak.[10] We discuss the duration of drain use in Chap. 5, "Postplacement Care."

Vasospasm and Delayed Cerebral Ischemia

Patients with aneurysmal subarachnoid hemorrhage (aSAH) are at increased risk of vasospasm and delayed cerebral ischemia (DCI). Most of the scientific community has moved away from equating angiographic vasospasm to DCI because of the low rate of co-occurrence. Although the

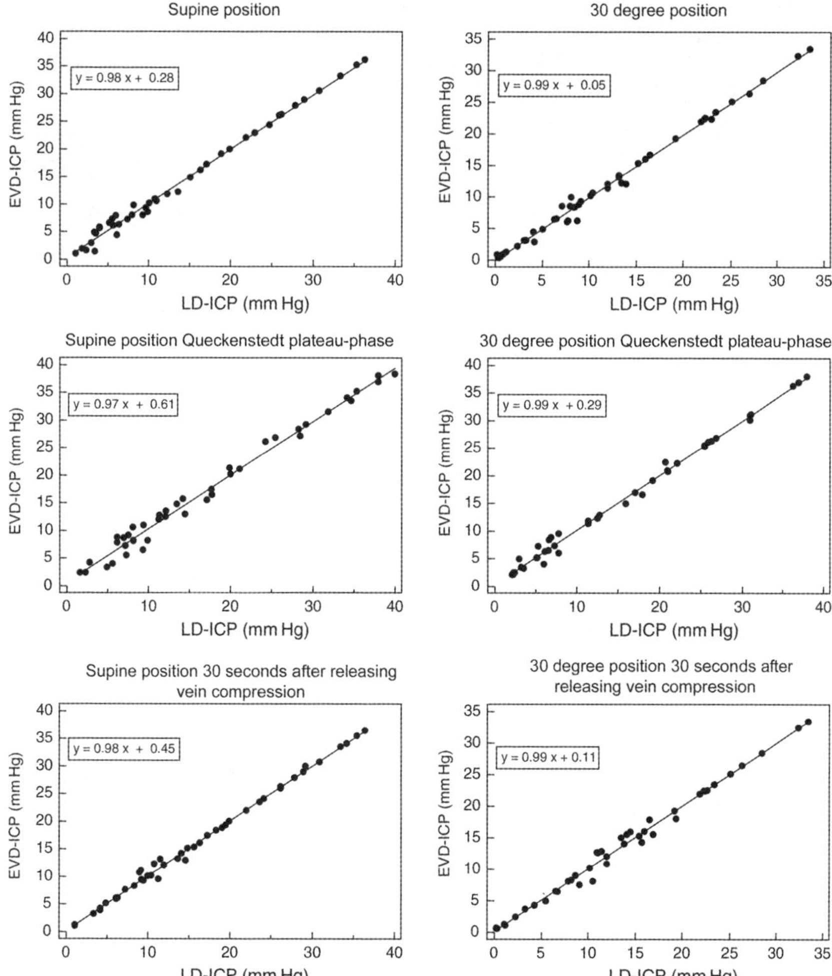

FIGURE 1.7. In a study of 43 patients with posthemorrhagic communicating hydrocephalus, Speck et al[7] found that intracranial pressure recordings from an external ventricular drain and a lumbar drain correlated nearly perfectly in a variety of positions, even with provocative maneuvers. EVD, external ventricular drain; ICP, intracranial pressure; LD, lumbar drain. *Used with permission from Speck V, Staykov D, Huttner HB, Sauer R, Schwab S, Bardutzky J. Lumbar catheter for monitoring of intracranial pressure in patients with post-hemorrhagic communicating hydrocephalus.* Neurocrit Care. *2011;14(2):208-215.*

cause of DCI has not yet been fully elucidated, evidence increasingly indicates that the type of drain may change the rate of DCI in patients with aSAH. One prospective randomized controlled trial that compared LD to standard medical management identified a significantly reduced occurrence of DCI in the LD group ($p = 0.02$) (Table 1.1).[11] One clinical trial has been initiated comparing EVD and LD head-to-head for this purpose

TABLE 1.1: PRIMARY INTENTION-TO-TREAT ANALYSIS OF 210 PATIENTS WITH SUBARACHNOID HEMORRHAGE TREATED WITH LUMBAR DRAINAGE OF CEREBROSPINAL FLUID*

Outcome Measure	Control Group ($n = 105$)	Study Group ($n = 105$)	Significance
Patients with DIND, No. (%)	37 (35.2)	22 (21.0)	$p = 0.02$
DIND in control group vs study group, OR (95% CI)		1.7 (1.1-2.6)	
Patients diagnosed with DIND and a persistent neurologic deficit at discharge, No. (%)	13 (12.4)	10 (9.5)	$p = 0.51$
Type of DIND			
Focal	21	9	
Altered consciousness	9	8	
Both	7	5	
Patients with radiologically confirmed infarct/patients imaged, No./Total (missing data)	31/91 (14)	23/94 (11)	$p = 0.15$
Patients with DIND and radiologically confirmed infarct/patients with DIND imaged, No./Total (missing data)	26/37 (0)	14/22 (0)	$p = 0.82$
Patients with DIND and radiologically established infarct, %	70	64	$p = 0.82$
Patients with mRS 0-2 at day 10, No. (%)	39 (37.5)	58 (55.2)	$p = 0.009$
Patients with mRS 0-2 at 6 months, No. (%)	83 (81.4)	81 (80.2)	$p = 0.83$
Patients dead at 6 months, No. (%)	5 (4.8)	4 (3.8)	$p > 0.99$
Patients requiring permanent CSF shunt, No. (%)	8 (7.6)	6 (5.7)	$p = 0.58$

CI, confidence interval; CSF, cerebrospinal fluid; DIND, delayed ischemic neurologic deficit; mRS, modified Rankin Scale; OR, odds ratio.

*Outcomes from the LUMAS trial showed significantly different rates of delayed ischemic neurologic deficit between patients in the experimental group managed by a lumbar drain and patients in the control group who underwent medical management of hydrocephalus.

Used with permission from Al-Tamimi et al, 2012.[11]

(Clinicaltrials.gov Identifier: NCT03065231). Given the data to date, we believe that LDs should be considered the first-line treatment for this population, assuming nonobstructive physiology.

EVDs have been used to deliver products to reduce DCI and improve outcomes. A phase 3 clinical trial of intraventricular nimodipine microparticles determined that nimodipine significantly reduced vasospasm ($p = 0.03$) but did not affect DCI or outcomes.[12] Another trial that used EVDs in patients with aSAH to clear intraventricular hemorrhage also used recombinant tissue-type plasminogen activator and head rotation.[13] Unfortunately, this phase 2 trial was not successful in reducing DCI, but a phase 3 trial is planned.[14] We (R.R. and colleagues) retrospectively investigated the benefit of intraventricular nicardipine for the prevention of vasospasm and likewise found no benefit (unpublished data).

Intraventricular Hemorrhage

Intraventricular hemorrhage is associated with a poor prognosis both in patients with aSAH and in patients with other forms of spontaneous intracranial hemorrhage; thus, it increases the need for a shunt. A major point of investigation has been whether to use EVDs to clear the hemorrhage. In the largest trial to date, CLEAR III, 1 mg of intraventricular alteplase administered every 8 hours did not meet the preset improvement in functional outcomes.[15] A 2017 randomized controlled trial showed a significant reduction in shunt dependency with a combined approach of intraventricular thrombolytics administered through the EVD and concurrent LD ($p = 0.007$).[16]

CNS Infection

The relatively impenetrable nature of the CNS due to the blood-brain barrier results in difficulty obtaining the necessary concentration of antibiotics to treat meningitis, ventriculitis, and cerebritis. Therefore, drains have been used to deliver these medications directly into the CNS. Reports exist on the administration via drains of antibiotics such as vancomycin,[17,18] gentamicin, tobramycin, amikacin,[18] colistin,[19] polymyxin B,[20] daptomycin, linezolid,[21] teicoplanin,[22] tigecycline,[23] amphotericin B,[24] and caspofungin.[25] However, most of these publications are case reports, and prospective trial data are scarce. The decision to insert a drain only for the purpose of treating a CNS infection or starting intraventricular therapy is case-dependent and should be made at the discretion of the treating team. Table 1.2 summarizes the medications and doses reported to have been administered via drains.[26-29]

TABLE 1.2: CENTRAL NERVOUS SYSTEM MEDICATIONS FOR INFECTIONS AS REPORTED IN THE MEDICAL LITERATURE

Medication	Dosage (Duration)	Organisms Treated	Toxicity Reported	Notes
Vancomycin	0.075-50 mg/d (1-90 days)	MRSA, *Enterococcus faecalis, Listeria monocytogenes, Propionibacterium acnes, Streptococcus sanguis, Staphylococcus epidermidis, Enterobacter cloacae, Escherichia coli, Klebsiella pneumoniae, Corynebacterium jeikeium*	Major: none Minor: nerve root irritation	One RCT: N = 27, 10 pts. on 10 mg/d for <10 days of prophylactic vancomycin and 17 pts. in control arm; none infected in vancomycin group; 47% in control[26]
Teicoplanin	5-20 mg/d (7-30 days)	MRSA, MRSE, *S. epidermidis, Enterococcus faecalis*	Major: none Minor: facial flushing	
Daptomycin	2.5-10 mg/d (7-30 days)	MRSE, VRE, *Enterococcus faecium*	Major: none Minor: transient fever	
Gentamicin	1-10 mg/d (3-35 days)	*K. pneumoniae, E. coli, Pseudomonas aeruginosa, Serratia marcescens, Sphingobacterium multivorum, S. intermedius, Streptococcus milleri, Acinetobacter baumannii, Proteus mirabilis, E. cloacae, S. epidermidis, Staphylococcus aureus, L. monocytogenes*	Major: lethargy Minor: none	75 mg, 3×/d: one report of patient who died from neurotoxicity[27]; intrathecal gentamycin combined with intravenous leads to complete treatment vs 33% relapse in IV-only group[28]
Amikacin	4-50 mg/d (3 days to 6 months)	*A. baumannii, E. coli, K. pneumoniae, P. aeruginosa,* multidrug-resistant *Mycobacterium tuberculosis, Citrobacter koseri, S. marcescens*	Major: hearing loss, seizures Minor: radiculopathy	

Tobramycin	5-20 mg/d (2-40 days)	*P. aeruginosa, K. pneumoniae, E. coli*	Major: none Minor: none	
Netilmicin	1-150 mg/d (10 days)	*S. aureus, S. epidermidis, K. pneumoniae, A. baumannii*	Major: none Minor: none	Often used in neonatal sepsis
Streptomycin	2-100 mg/d (4-33 days)	*Mycobacterium tuberculosis*, VRE, *Haemophilus influenzae*	Major: respiratory failure, seizures, coma, death Minor: nausea	Largely abandoned because of severe side effect profile
Penicillin	Depends on class	*S. aureus, S. epidermidis, H. influenzae, E. coli*	Major: seizures Minor: none	Largely abandoned because of severe side effect profile
Lincomycin	2 mg/d (5-9 days)	*S. aureus, S. hemolyticus, Enterococcus faecalis, Streptococcus pyogenes*	Major: none Minor: none	Older antibiotic
Cephalosporin	25-100 mg/d (3-19 days)	*Klebsiella enterobacter, S. epidermidis, S. aureus, Streptococcus pneumoniae, Corynebacterium diphtheriae, Streptococcus intermedius*	Major: seizures, death Minor: vomiting	Largely abandoned because of severe side effect profile
Erythromycin	3-25 mg/d (5-12 days)	*Flavobacterium meningosepticum*	Major: none Minor: none	Older antibiotic
Polymyxin B	2000-100,000 units/d (5-30 days)	Multi-drug resistant *A. baumannii, K. pneumoniae, Pseudomonas pyocyanea*	Major: none Minor: meningeal irritation	

(Continued)

TABLE 1.2: CENTRAL NERVOUS SYSTEM MEDICATIONS FOR INFECTIONS AS REPORTED IN THE MEDICAL LITERATURE *(Continued)*

Medication	Dosage (Duration)	Organisms Treated	Toxicity Reported	Notes
Colistin	12,500-500,000 IU/d (2-40 days)	Multi-drug resistant *A. baumannii, P. aeruginosa, K. pneumoniae, Achromobacter xylosoxidans, Acinetobacter lwoffii, Enterobacter cloacae, S. epidermidis, S. hemolyticus,* NDM-1 *K. pneumoniae*	Major: rare nephrotoxicity or seizures Minor: meningeal irritation	
Chloramphenicol	0.1 mg-50 mg/d (3-35 days)	VRE, *S. aureus, E. coli, Salmonella,* group B *Streptococcus*	Major: none Minor: none	Risk of aplastic anemia (not shown with CSF injection)
Rifampin	2-5 mg/d (7-50 days)	*F. meningosepticum, Mycobacterium tuberculosis*	Major: none Minor: transient jaundice	Replaced as drug of choice by isoniazid
Isoniazid	5-100 mg every 1-3 days until symptoms improve	*Mycobacterium tuberculosis*	Major: aphasia, hemiplegia or quadriplegia, optic atrophy, transient herniation, hepatoxicity Minor: none	Significant side effects; use with caution

CSF, cerebrospinal fluid; IV, intravenous; RCT, randomized controlled trial; MRSA, methicillin-resistant *Staphylococcus aureus*; MRSE, methicillin-resistant *Staphylococcus epidermidis*; VRE: vancomycin-resistant enterococci.

Data from Mrowczynski et al.[29]

Other Uses

LDs have also been proposed as adjunct treatments in patients with traumatic spinal cord injury and thoracoabdominal aorta surgery.[30-32] The rationale for the use of an LD in such cases rests on the concept of spinal cord perfusion pressure (SCPP), which involves the balance of mean arterial pressure (MAP) and intrathecal pressure (ITP). SCPP can be modeled using the equation:

$$SCPP = MAP - ITP$$

Removing excess CSF results in a reduction of ITP. With maintenance or increase of MAP, the SCPP is improved, thus preventing ischemic complications in the spinal cord.[33] ITP monitoring has been used both during surgery to establish that adequate decompression has been achieved and postoperatively to register decreases in SCPP that are missed by MAP monitoring alone.[34] Because LDs have a reasonable safety profile and provide meaningful data in the management of both of these patient populations, we are in favor of their use in such cases.

LDs have also been proposed for use in patients with elevated refractory ICP. In a small prospective study of eight patients with EVDs who continued to have medically refractory ICP despite placement of the EVD, the authors found that the use of an LD led to a significant decrease in ICP to normal levels ($p < 0.05$), with no complications, and to a reduction in medical therapies.[35] This small prospective study reinforces the possible overdramatization in the medical literature of the fear of herniation and suggests that the vigilant use of LDs can be safe even in traditionally contraindicated cases.

ABBREVIATIONS

aSAH, aneurysmal subarachnoid hemorrhage

CNS, central nervous system

CSF, cerebrospinal fluid

DCI, delayed cerebral ischemia

EVD, external ventricular drain

ICP, intracranial pressure

ITP, intrathecal pressure

LD, lumbar drain

MAP, mean arterial pressure

SCPP, spinal cord perfusion pressure

REFERENCES

1. Tomycz LD, Hale AT, George TM. Emerging insights and new perspectives on the nature of hydrocephalus. *Pediatr Neurosurg.* 2017;52(6):361-368. doi:10.1159/000484173.
2. Brinker T, Stopa E, Morrison J, Klinge P. A new look at cerebrospinal fluid circulation. *Fluids Barriers CNS.* 2014;11:10. doi:10.1186/2045-8118-11-10.
3. Bulat M, Klarica M. Recent insights into a new hydrodynamics of the cerebrospinal fluid. *Brain Res Rev.* 2011;65(2):99-112. doi:10.1016/j.brainresrev.2010.08.002.
4. Oreskovic D, Klarica M. The formation of cerebrospinal fluid: nearly a hundred years of interpretations and misinterpretations. *Brain Res Rev.* 2010;64(2):241-262. doi:10.1016/j.brainresrev.2010.04.006.
5. Panni P, Donofrio CA, Barzaghi LR, et al. Safety and feasibility of lumbar drainage in the management of poor grade aneurysmal subarachnoid hemorrhage. *J Clin Neurosci.* 2019;64:64-70. doi:10.1016/j.jocn.2019.04.010.
6. Cushing H. *Studies in Intracranial Physiology & Surgery: The Third Circulation, the Hypophysics, the Gliomas.* London: H. Milford, Oxford University Press; 1926.
7. Speck V, Staykov D, Huttner HB, Sauer R, Schwab S, Bardutzky J. Lumbar catheter for monitoring of intracranial pressure in patients with post-hemorrhagic communicating hydrocephalus. *Neurocrit Care.* 2011;14(2):208-215. doi:10.1007/s12028-010-9459-6.
8. Zwagerman NT, Wang EW, Shin SS, et al. Does lumbar drainage reduce postoperative cerebrospinal fluid leak after endoscopic endonasal skull base surgery? A prospective, randomized controlled trial. *J Neurosurg.* 2018:1-7. doi:10.3171/2018.4.JNS172447.
9. Khan R, Sajjad M, Khan AA, et al. Comparison of lumbar drain insertion and conservative management in the treatment of traumatic CSF rhinorrhoea. *J Ayub Med Coll Abbottabad.* 2019;31(3):441-444.
10. Tunkel AR, Hasbun R, Bhimraj A, et al. 2017 Infectious Diseases Society of America's clinical practice guidelines for healthcare-associated ventriculitis and meningitis. *Clin Infect Dis.* 2017;64(6):e34-e65. doi:10.1093/cid/ciw861.
11. Al-Tamimi YZ, Bhargava D, Feltbower RG, et al. Lumbar drainage of cerebrospinal fluid after aneurysmal subarachnoid hemorrhage: a prospective, randomized, controlled trial (LUMAS). *Stroke.* Mar 2012;43(3):677-682. doi:10.1161/STROKEAHA.111.625731.
12. Carlson AP, Hanggi D, Wong GK, et al. Single-dose intraventricular nimodipine microparticles versus oral nimodipine for aneurysmal subarachnoid hemorrhage. *Stroke.* 2020;51(4):1142-1149. doi:10.1161/STROKEAHA.119.027396.
13. Etminan N, Beseoglu K, Eicker SO, Turowski B, Steiger HJ, Hanggi D. Prospective, randomized, open-label phase II trial on concomitant intraventricular fibrinolysis and low-frequency rotation after severe subarachnoid hemorrhage. *Stroke.* 2013;44(8):2162-2168. doi:10.1161/STROKEAHA.113.001790.
14. Gaberel T, Gakuba C, Fournel F, et al. FIVHeMA: Intraventricular fibrinolysis versus external ventricular drainage alone in aneurysmal subarachnoid hemorrhage: a randomized controlled trial. *Neurochirurgie.* 2019;65(1):14-19. doi:10.1016/j.neuchi.2018.11.004.
15. Hanley DF, Lane K, McBee N, et al. Thrombolytic removal of intraventricular haemorrhage in treatment of severe stroke: results of the randomised, multicentre, multiregion, placebo-controlled CLEAR III trial. *Lancet.* 2017;389(10069):603-611. doi:10.1016/S0140-6736(16)32410-2.
16. Staykov D, Kuramatsu JB, Bardutzky J, et al. Efficacy and safety of combined intraventricular fibrinolysis with lumbar drainage for prevention of permanent shunt

dependency after intracerebral hemorrhage with severe ventricular involvement: a randomized trial and individual patient data meta-analysis. *Ann Neurol.* 2017;81(1): 93-103. doi:10.1002/ana.24834.

17. Pfausler B, Haring HP, Kampfl A, Wissel J, Schober M, Schmutzhard E. Cerebrospinal fluid (CSF) pharmacokinetics of intraventricular vancomycin in patients with staphylococcal ventriculitis associated with external CSF drainage. *Clin Infect Dis.* 1997;25(3):733-735. doi:10.1086/513756.

18. Pfausler B, Spiss H, Beer R, et al. Treatment of staphylococcal ventriculitis associated with external cerebrospinal fluid drains: a prospective randomized trial of intravenous compared with intraventricular vancomycin therapy. *J Neurosurg.* 2003;98(5):1040-1044. doi:10.3171/jns.2003.98.5.1040.

19. Imberti R, Cusato M, Accetta G, et al. Pharmacokinetics of colistin in cerebrospinal fluid after intraventricular administration of colistin methanesulfonate. *Antimicrob Agents Chemother.* 2012;56(8):4416-4421. doi:10.1128/AAC.00231-12.

20. Pan S, Huang X, Wang Y, et al. Efficacy of intravenous plus intrathecal/intracerebral ventricle injection of polymyxin B for post-neurosurgical intracranial infections due to MDR/XDR *Acinectobacter baumannii*: a retrospective cohort study. *Antimicrob Resist Infect Control.* 2018;7:8. doi:10.1186/s13756-018-0305-5.

21. Mueller SW, Kiser TH, Anderson TA, Neumann RT. Intraventricular daptomycin and intravenous linezolid for the treatment of external ventricular-drain-associated ventriculitis due to vancomycin-resistant *Enterococcus faecium*. *Ann Pharmacother.* 2012;46(12):e35. doi:10.1345/aph.1R412.

22. Beenen LF, Touw DJ, Hekker TA, Haring DA. Pharmacokinetics of intraventricularly administered teicoplanin in *Staphylococci ventriculitis*. *Pharm World Sci.* 2000;22(4):127-129. doi:10.1023/a:1008719806949.

23. Wu Y, Chen K, Zhao J, Wang Q, Zhou J. Intraventricular administration of tigecycline for the treatment of multidrug-resistant bacterial meningitis after craniotomy: a case report. *J Chemother.* 2018;30(1):49-52. doi:10.1080/1120009X.2017.1338846.

24. Toprak D, Ocal Demir S, Kadayifci EK, Turel O, Soysal A, Bakir M. Recurrent *Candida albicans ventriculitis* treated with intraventricular liposomal amphotericin B. *Case Rep Infect Dis.* 2015;2015:340725. doi:10.1155/2015/340725.

25. Williams JR, Tenforde MW, Chan JD, Ko A, Graham SM. Safety and clinical response of intraventricular caspofungin for *Scedosporium apiospermum* complex central nervous system infection. *Med Mycol Case Rep.* 2016;13:1-4. doi:10.1016/j.mmcr.2016.07.003.

26. Morales-García VD G-MR, Tamez-Montes D, Martínez-Ponce LA. Efficacy of prophylactic intraventricular vancomycin in patients with ventriculostomy. *Arch Neurosci.* 2005;10(3):128-132.

27. Watanabe I, Hodges GR, Dworzack DL, Kepes JJ, Duensing GF. Neurotoxicity of intrathecal gentamicin: a case report and experimental study. *Ann Neurol.* Dec 1978;4(6):564-572. doi:10.1002/ana.410040618.

28. Tangden T, Enblad P, Ullberg M, Sjolin J. Neurosurgical gram-negative bacillary ventriculitis and meningitis: a retrospective study evaluating the efficacy of intraventricular gentamicin therapy in 31 consecutive cases. *Clin Infect Dis.* 2011;52(11):1310-1316. doi:10.1093/cid/cir197.

29. Mrowczynski OD, Langan ST, Rizk EB. Intra-cerebrospinal fluid antibiotics to treat central nervous system infections: a review and update. *Clin Neurol Neurosurg.* 2018;170:140-158. doi:10.1016/j.clineuro.2018.05.007.

30. Yue JK, Hemmerle DD, Winkler EA, et al. Clinical implementation of novel spinal cord perfusion pressure protocol in acute traumatic spinal cord injury at U.S. Level I Trauma Center: TRACK-SCI Study. *World Neurosurg.* 2020;133:e391-e396. doi:10.1016/j.wneu.2019.09.044.

31. Khan NR, Smalley Z, Nesvick CL, Lee SL, Michael LM 2nd. The use of lumbar drains in preventing spinal cord injury following thoracoabdominal aortic aneurysm repair: an updated systematic review and meta-analysis. *J Neurosurg Spine.* 2016;25(3):383-393. doi:10.3171/2016.1.SPINE151199.

32. Coselli JS, LeMaire SA, Koksoy C, Schmittling ZC, Curling PE. Cerebrospinal fluid drainage reduces paraplegia after thoracoabdominal aortic aneurysm repair: results of a randomized clinical trial. *J Vasc Surg.* 2002;35(4):631-639. doi:10.1067/mva.2002.122024.

33. Saadoun S, Papadopoulos MC. Targeted perfusion therapy in spinal cord trauma. *Neurotherapeutics.* 2020;17(2):511-521. doi:10.1007/s13311-019-00820-6.

34. Kwon BK, Curt A, Belanger LM, et al. Intrathecal pressure monitoring and cerebrospinal fluid drainage in acute spinal cord injury: a prospective randomized trial. *J Neurosurg Spine.* 2009;10(3):181-193. doi:10.3171/2008.10.SPINE08217.

35. Murad A, Ghostine S, Colohan AR. Controlled lumbar drainage in medically refractory increased intracranial pressure: a safe and effective treatment. *Acta Neurochir Suppl.* 2008;102:89-91. doi:10.1007/978-3-211-85578-2_18.

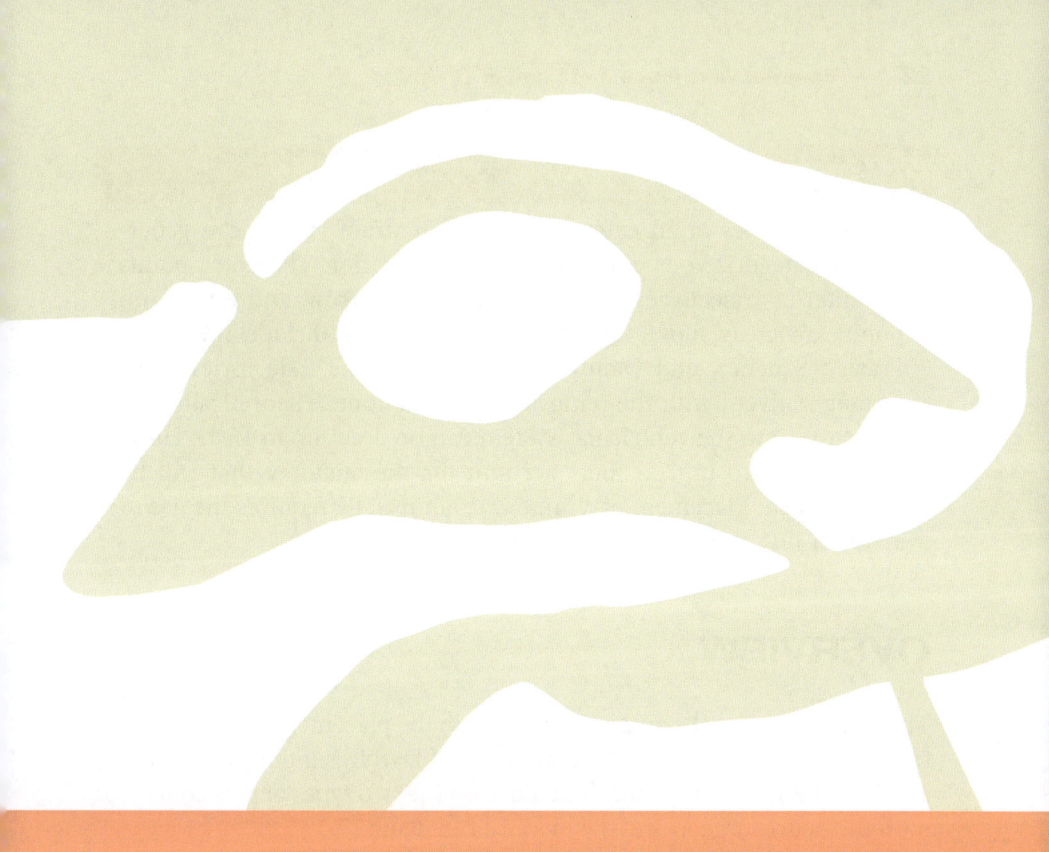

CHAPTER 2

Anatomy

CHAPTER SUMMARY

The trajectories of an external ventricular drain (EVD) can generally be categorized as either anterior or posterior. The entry points for anterior trajectories include the Kocher, Barrow, and Kaufmann points, whereas those for posterior trajectories include the Keen, Frazier, Sanchez, and Dandy points. These same trajectories apply intraoperatively, with the removal of cranial bone. Theoretically, any trajectory into the ventricular system can be used for an EVD. However, the neurosurgeon must account for the anatomy that will be transgressed. Placement of a lumbar drain usually requires the use of a Tuffier line at the L4-L5 intervertebral space.

OVERVIEW

This chapter covers the anatomy involved in the placement of external ventricular drains (EVDs) and lumbar drains (LDs). It is intended to provide a rationale for drain use and a reference on the two types of procedures for both the neurosurgeon and the medical care team.

ANATOMY OF VENTRICULAR ACCESS

Technically, any point on the scalp can be used as a straight-line entrance into the ventricles. The process is not this simple, though, because the brain that is transgressed is eloquent; therefore, the path with the least potential damage must be chosen. Several named points have historically been proven to be safe sites for access (Table 2.1). We invite the readers to review an excellent summary by Morone et al.[1] of these named points.

ANTERIOR APPROACHES

The Kocher, Barrow, and Kaufmann points are three of the entry points for anterior trajectories for EVD placement. The most common entry point for an anterior trajectory is the Kocher point, which has been described in various ways. In the anterior-posterior dimension, some neurosurgeons mark the Kocher point 10 to 11 cm up from the nasion, whereas others use a point that is 25% of the distance from the nasion

TABLE 2.1: OVERVIEW OF EXTERNAL VENTRICULAR DRAIN ACCESS POINTS AND TRAJECTORIES

Point Name	Landmarks and Trajectories
Anterior approaches	
Kocher	10 to 11 cm from the nasion and 2 to 3 cm from the midline at the midpupillary line, then to the ipsilateral medial canthus, nasion, or contralateral medial canthus and the ipsilateral external auditory canal to a depth of 5 to 6 cm
Barrow	1 cm anterior and 1 cm superior to the anterior-superior attachment of the pinna, then perpendicular to the temporal squama to a depth of 4 cm
Kaufmann	5 cm superior to the nasion and 3 cm lateral to the midline, then to the midline and 3 cm superior to the inion to a depth of 5 to 6 cm
Posterior approaches	
Keen	2.5 to 3 cm superior and posterior to the pinna of the ear, then to the ipsilateral trigone of the lateral ventricle perpendicular to the bone to a depth of 4 to 5 cm
Frazier	6 cm above the inion and 3 to 4 cm lateral to the midline or lambda, the trajectory is directed medially and superiorly to a point that is 4 cm above the contralateral medial canthus to a depth of 5 cm
Sanchez	6 cm above the inion and 3 to 4 cm lateral to the midline or lambda, then just lateral from the midline at 5° and 30° inferiorly
Dandy	3 cm above the inion and 2 cm from the midline, then superiorly and medially to 3 cm above the nasion to a depth of 5 cm

to the external occipital protuberance because it is applicable to any head size (Fig. 2.1A). The most important consideration is to be at least 1 cm anterior to the coronal suture to avoid the motor strip.[2–4] In the lateral dimension, the reported values are 2 to 3 cm off the midline or at the midpupillary line (Fig. 2.1B).[2,3] The catheter is then advanced until the lateral ventricle is entered by using the external landmarks of the ipsilateral medial canthus, the nasion or contralateral medial canthus, and the ipsilateral external auditory canal.[5] The lateral ventricle is usually encountered at 5 to 6 cm, and we allow the catheter to go no deeper than 7 cm. This trajectory is most often performed on the right side because the right frontal lobe is less likely to be eloquent for speech, but it can also be performed on the left. The catheter will enter through either the superior or middle frontal gyrus, likely avoiding the Broca area even on the left.

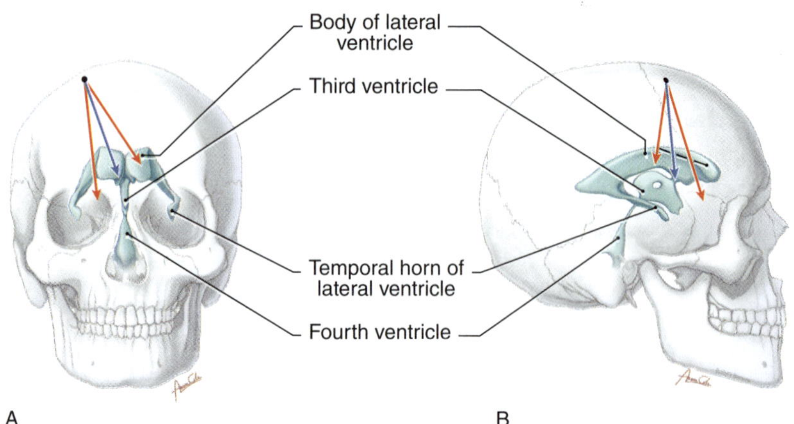

A   B

FIGURE 2.1. Kocher point. **A.** Anterior view, with correct (*blue arrow*) and incorrect (*red arrows*) trajectories. **B.** Lateral view, with correct (*blue arrow*) and incorrect (*red arrows*) trajectories. The entrance point should be 1 cm anterior to the coronal suture, roughly at the midpupillary line. The trajectory should aim for the ipsilateral medial canthus and tragus just in front of the external auditory canal, which places the terminal point in the ipsilateral foramen of Monro. A trajectory that is too lateral risks injury to the ipsilateral internal capsule and one that is too medial risks injury to the fornix and contralateral internal capsule. Too posterior a trajectory increases risk to the thalamus. The ventricle should be encountered in almost all cases within 5 to 6 cm; thus, advancing deeper than 7 cm increases the risk to deep structures and arteries.

The midline is avoided to protect the sagittal sinus and bridging veins. A trajectory that is too lateral will place the catheter in the caudate nucleus, the internal capsule, or the globus pallidus. A trajectory that is too posterior and lateral will lead to the thalamus.

A second anterior approach, the Barrow point, involves access to the anterior temporal horn of the lateral ventricle.[6] This point is located roughly 1 cm anterior to and 1 cm superior to the anterior-superior attachment of the pinna (Fig. 2.2). The trajectory from the Barrow point is perpendicular to the temporal squama. The catheter is advanced 4 cm until it reaches the temporal horn of the lateral ventricle. The pathway goes through the middle temporal gyrus, which puts the optic radiations at some risk. Likewise, too deep an insertion places the brainstem at risk.

A third anterior entry point is the Kaufmann point.[7] This point is located 5 cm superior to the nasion and 3 cm lateral to the midline (Fig. 2.3). The catheter is advanced no more than 7 cm and is advanced in the direction of the midline and a point that is 3 cm superior to the inion and advanced to the lateral ventricle. The catheter will transgress the superior frontal gyrus. This approach can be performed on either side. Too lateral a trajectory risks injury to the basal ganglia and internal capsule.

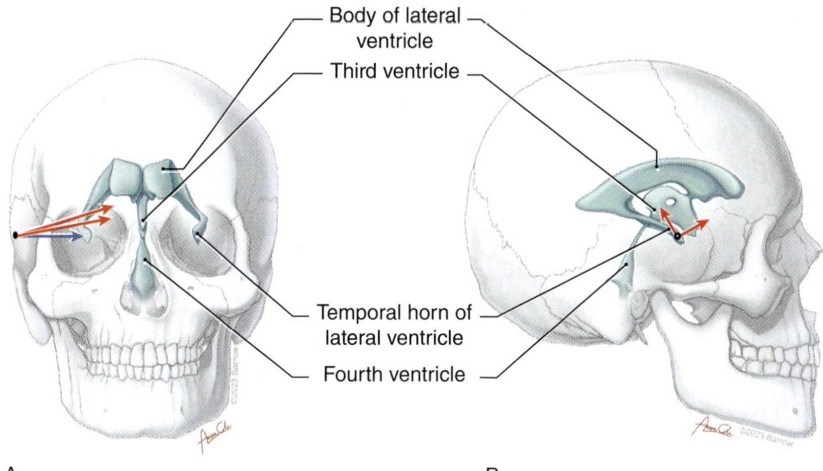

FIGURE 2.2. Barrow point. **A.** Anterior view, with correct (*blue arrow*) and incorrect (*red arrows*) trajectories. **B.** Lateral view, with incorrect trajectories (*red arrows*); in this view, the correct trajectory is 90° to the lateral surface and is not shown. Entrance is approximately 1 cm anterior and superior to the anterior-superior attachment of the pinna. Entering perpendicular to the sagittal plane and advancing to 4 cm should advance the tip of the catheter into the temporal horn of the lateral ventricle. Advancing too deep will place the brainstem at risk. Aiming superiorly will risk injury to the internal capsule.

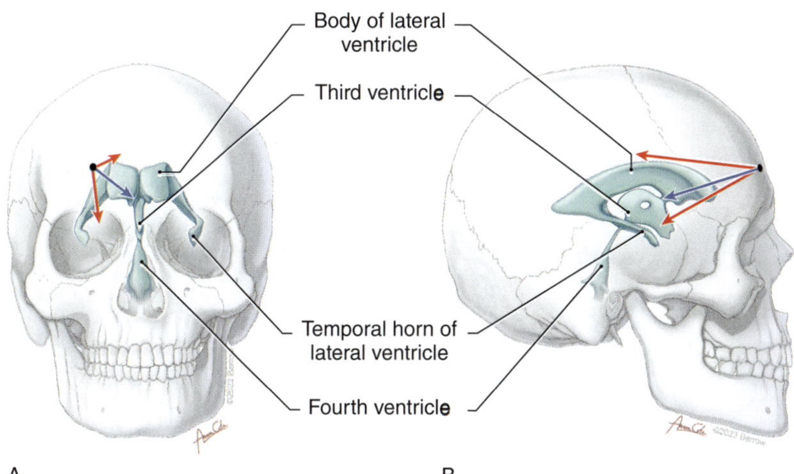

FIGURE 2.3. Kaufmann point. **A.** Anterior view, with correct (*blue arrow*) and incorrect (*red arrows*) trajectories. **B.** Lateral view, with correct (*blue arrow*) and incorrect (*red arrows*) trajectories. The entry point is on the forehead, approximately 5 cm superior to the nasion and at the midpupillary line. The trajectory is aimed at the midline and a point that is approximately 3 cm above the inion until it reaches the frontal horn of lateral ventricle. Too lateral a trajectory will risk injury to the internal capsule and basal ganglia.

POSTERIOR APPROACHES

The Keen, Frazier, Sanchez, and Dandy points are four common entry points for posterior trajectories for EVD placement. The Keen point is located 2.5 to 3 cm superior and posterior to the pinna of the ear.[8] The catheter is then advanced 4 to 5 cm to enter the ipsilateral trigone of the lateral ventricle by staying perpendicular to the skull at the entry point (Fig. 2.4). This trajectory can be accessed on either side but requires side-dependent positioning, unlike with the previous Kocher and Kaufmann access points. This trajectory will transgress through the supramarginal or angular gyrus, thus putting more eloquent brain at risk.

The second entry point for a posterior trajectory is the Frazier point, which is located 6 cm above the inion and 3 to 4 cm lateral to the midline in the region of the lambdoid suture.[1] The trajectory is directed medially and superiorly to a a point that is 4 cm above the contralateral medial canthus (Fig. 2.5). The catheter is advanced at least 5 cm to enter the body of the ipsilateral lateral ventricle. This trajectory will transgress the superior parietal lobule. Deviation laterally will place the catheter in the posterior limb of the internal capsule or thalamus. This approach can be performed on either side. A modification of this trajectory begins at the Sanchez point, and targets the temporal horn instead of the body

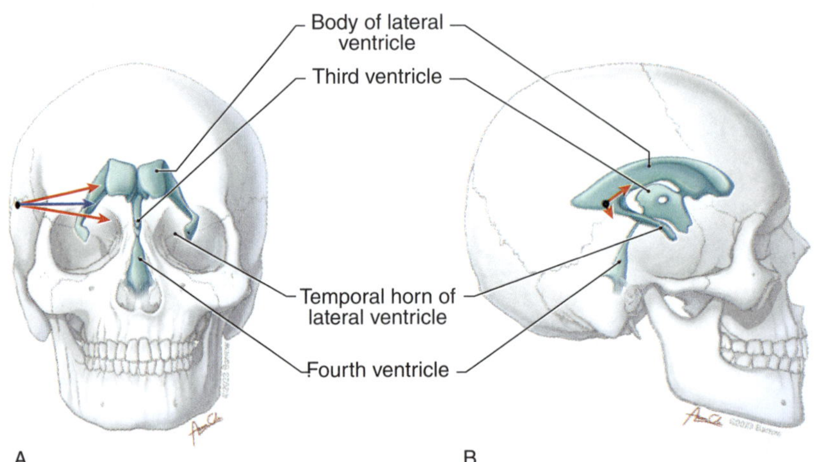

FIGURE 2.4. Keen point. **A.** Anterior view, with correct (*blue arrow*) and incorrect (*red arrows*) trajectories. **B.** Lateral view, with incorrect trajectories (*red arrows*); in this view, the correct trajectory is 90° to the lateral spurface and, therefore, is not shown. Entrance is approximately 3 cm superior and posterior to the pinna of the ear. The trajectory is perpendicular to the sagittal plane, and the catheter is advanced no more than 5 cm to enter the ventricular trigone. A trajectory that is too inferior or anterior risks injury to the thalamus, whereas a trajectory that is too posterior risks injury to the optic radiations.

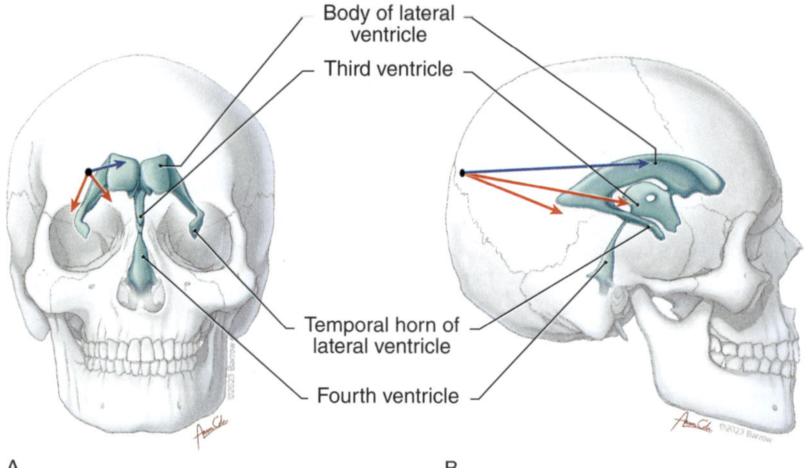

FIGURE 2.5. Frazier point. **A.** Posterior to anterior view, with correct (*blue arrow*) and incorrect (*red arrows*) trajectories. **B.** Lateral view, with correct (*blue arrow*) and incorrect (*red arrows*) trajectories. Entrance is approximately 6 cm above the inion and 3 cm lateral to the midline. The trajectory is directed medially and superiorly to a point 4 cm above the contralateral medial canthus. The catheter is advanced to 5 cm. Deviating laterally will risk injury to the internal capsule and thalamus.

of the lateral ventricle.[9] The entry point is the same, but the catheter is directed 5° laterally and 30° inferiorly (Fig. 2.6).

The fourth entry point for a posterior trajectory is the Dandy point, which is located 3 cm above the inion and 2 cm from the midline.[1] The trajectory is directed superiorly and medially to a point 3 cm above the nasion (Fig. 2.7). The catheter is advanced 5 cm until it reaches the body of the lateral ventricle. The trajectory from the Dandy point is more likely to pass through the occipital lobe than the trajectory from the Frazier point, risking injury to the optic radiations. This approach can also be performed on either side.

INTRAOPERATIVE ACCESS

A number of ventricular access points have been described for intraoperative use. These points are used to decompress the brain during surgery to make visualization easier. Once a catheter has been passed, it can be left in place and made to exit through the craniotomy for use after the surgery.

For a pterional, frontotemporal, or orbitozygomatic craniotomy, access to the ventricles can be obtained intracranially from points on the surface of the exposed brain. The Paine point is located 2.5 cm above the orbital roof and 2.5 cm anterior to the sylvian fissure.[10] The trajectory from the Paine

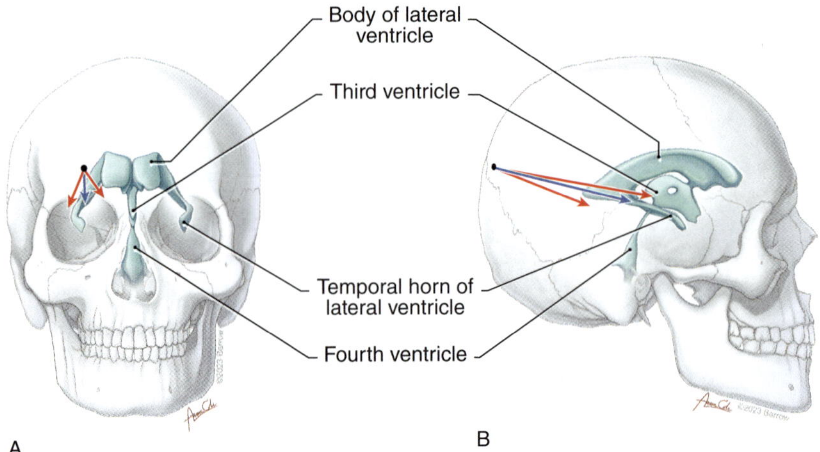

FIGURE 2.6. Sanchez point. **A.** Posterior to anterior view, with correct (*blue arrow*) and incorrect (*red arrows*) trajectories. **B.** Lateral view, with correct (*blue arrow*) and incorrect (*red arrows*) trajectories. The entry point is the same as that for the Frazier point; however, the trajectory is for the temporal part of the lateral ventricle, aiming approximately for the ipsilateral pupil. The catheter is advanced 5 cm. Deviating superiorly will place it in the lateral ventricle or thalamus.

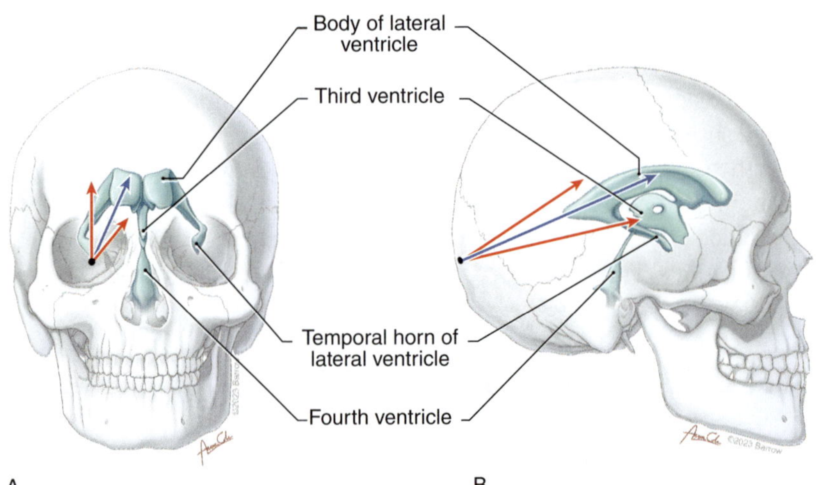

FIGURE 2.7. Dandy point. **A.** Posterior to anterior view, with correct (*blue arrow*) and incorrect (*red arrows*) trajectories. **B.** Lateral view, with correct (*blue arrow*) and incorrect (*red arrows*) trajectories. Entrance is located 3 cm above the inion and 2 cm from the midline. The trajectory is superior and medial to a point 3 cm above the nasion and is advanced 5 cm. Too inferior or lateral a trajectory will place the catheter in the thalamus or internal capsule. A trajectory that is too superior will place it into the sensory and motor tracts.

point is directly perpendicular to the brain, and the catheter is inserted to a depth of 4 to 5 cm until the frontal horn of the lateral ventricle is entered. This location is approximately in the inferior frontal gyrus, which puts the Broca area, the caudate nucleus, and the basal ganglia at risk. If the trajectory is positioned too posteriorly, it puts the thalamus at risk. Given these risks, two modifications have been proposed. Park and Hamm[11] proposed moving the intracranial entry point 2 cm anterior to the Paine point. Hyun et al[12] proposed moving the entry point 2 cm superior to the entrance point to avoid these critical structures.

After a supraorbital craniotomy, Menovsky et al[13] proposed a frontal approach for intracranial access to the ventricles. The catheter trajectory is 45° toward the midline and 20° superiorly from the orbitomeatal line, and the catheter is passed to a depth of 5 to 6 cm.

Theoretically, as with extracranial scalp-based entry points, any craniotomy exposes a surface of brain that lends itself to accessing the ventricles intracranially. The question becomes how much transgression of eloquent brain is acceptable.

ANATOMY OF LUMBAR ACCESS

The anatomy in the lumbar region is arguably more straightforward than the cranial anatomy. The most important factor to consider in placing an LD is the location of the conus medullaris.

The normal range of the bottom of the human spinal cord has been documented as being between T12 and L3, and it reaches this level in each person by the age of 2 years.[14] In a magnetic resonance imaging (MRI) study of 504 adult patients without spinal pathology, the position of the conus medullaris was shown to have a normal distribution of termination from the lower third of T12 to the upper third of L3.[14] Spinal pathology does not appear to play a role in the location of the conus. In an MRI study of 234 patients with spinal stenosis, the location of the conus also followed a normal distribution, from the middle third of T12 to the upper third of L3.[15] Age appears to be the main factor that determines the location of the conus. In an MRI study of 350 children ages 1 month to 20 years, the lowest location of the conus was at the L3-L4 space in a group of 6- to 12-month-old patients.[16]

For assessments of the anatomy of the lumbar spine for drain placement, the primary measurement is the Tuffier line, a line joining the two highest points of the iliac crests. This line is used to approximate the interspinous segment where entrance can be made. MRI in 690 patients showed that the position of the Tuffier line relative to the spine ranged from the L3-L4 intervertebral space to the L5-S1 intervertebral space, with a median location at the L4-L5 intervertebral space.[17] The distance between the Tuffier line and the conus is shorter in older adults and female patients, but, importantly, it never crosses the conus medullaris. Therefore, given the low probability of the conus existing at this level, lumbar puncture is safe, certainly up to the L3-L4 space, and it can even be considered at the L2-L3 intervertebral space when prior levels have failed. The distance between the skin and intervertebral space depends on the body habitus.

ABBREVIATIONS

EVD, external ventricular drain

LD, lumbar drain

MRI, magnetic resonance imaging

REFERENCES

1. Morone PJ, Dewan MC, Zuckerman SL, Tubbs RS, Singer RJ. Craniometrics and ventricular access: a review of Kocher's, Kaufman's, Paine's, Menovksy's, Tubbs', Keen's, Frazier's, Dandy's, and Sanchez's points. *Oper Neurosurg (Hagerstown)*. 2020;18(5): 461-469. doi:10.1093/ons/opz194.
2. Ghajar JB. A guide for ventricular catheter placement. Technical note. *J Neurosurg*. 1985;63(6):985-986. doi:10.3171/jns.1985.63.6.0985.
3. McWilliam RC, Stephenson JB. Rapid bedside technique for intracranial pressure monitoring. *Lancet*. 1984;2(8394):73-75. doi:10.1016/s0140-6736(84)90244-7.
4. Keen WW, Da Costa JC. *Surgery: Its Principles and Practice*. Philadelphia, PA: W.B. Saunders Company; 1908.
5. Amoo M, Henry J, Javadpour M. Common trajectories for freehand frontal ventriculostomy: a systematic review. *World Neurosurg*. 2021;146:292-297. doi:10.1016/j. wneu.2020.11.065.
6. Bohl MA, Almefty KK, Nakaji P. Defining a standardized approach for the bedside insertion of temporal horn external ventricular drains: procedure development and case series. *Neurosurgery*. 2016;79(2):296-304. doi:10.1227/NEU.0000000000001164.
7. Kaufmann GE, Clark K. Emergency frontal twist drill ventriculostomy. Technical note. *J Neurosurg*. 1970;33(2):226-227. doi:10.3171/jns.1970.33.2.0226.
8. Keen WW. Surgery of the lateral ventricles of the brain. *Lancet*. 1890;136(3498):553-555.
9. Sanchez JJ, Rincon-Torroella J, Prats-Galino A, et al. New endoscopic route to the temporal horn of the lateral ventricle: surgical simulation and morphometric assessment. *J Neurosurg*. 2014;121(3):751-759. doi:10.3171/2014.5.JNS132309.
10. Paine JT, Batjer HH, Samson D. Intraoperative ventricular puncture. *Neurosurgery*. 1988;22(6 Pt 1):1107-1109. doi:10.1227/00006123-198806010-00027.

11. Park J, Hamm IS. Revision of Paine's technique for intraoperative ventricular puncture. *Surg Neurol.* 2008;70(5):503-508; discussion 508. doi:10.1016/j.surneu.2007.09.018.

12. Hyun SJ, Suk JS, Kwon JT, Kim YB. Novel entry point for intraoperative ventricular puncture during the transsylvian approach. *Acta Neurochir (Wien).* 2007;149(10): 1049-1051; discussion 1051. doi:10.1007/s00701-007-1281-3.

13. Menovsky T, De Vries J, Wurzer JA, Grotenhuis JA. Intraoperative ventricular puncture during supraorbital craniotomy via an eyebrow incision. Technical note. *J Neurosurg.* 2006;105(3):485-486. doi:10.3171/jns.2006.105.3.485.

14. Saifuddin A, Burnett SJ, White J. The variation of position of the conus medullaris in an adult population. A magnetic resonance imaging study. *Spine (Phila Pa 1976).* 1998;23(13):1452-1456. doi:10.1097/00007632-199807010-00005.

15. Ba Z, Zhao W, Wu D, Huang Y, Kan H. MRI study of the position of the conus medullaris in patients with lumbar spinal stenosis. *Orthopedics.* 2012;35(6):e899-e902. doi:10.3928/01477447-20120525-31.

16. Jung JY, Kim EH, Song IK, Lee JH, Kim HS, Kim JT. The influence of age on positions of the conus medullaris, Tuffier's line, dural sac, and sacrococcygeal membrane in infants, children, adolescents, and young adults. *Paediatr Anaesth.* 2016;26(12): 1172-1178. doi:10.1111/pan.12998.

17. Kim JT, Bahk JH, Sung J. Influence of age and sex on the position of the conus medullaris and Tuffier's line in adults. *Anesthesiology.* 2003;99(6):1359-1363. doi:10.1097/00000542-200312000-00018.

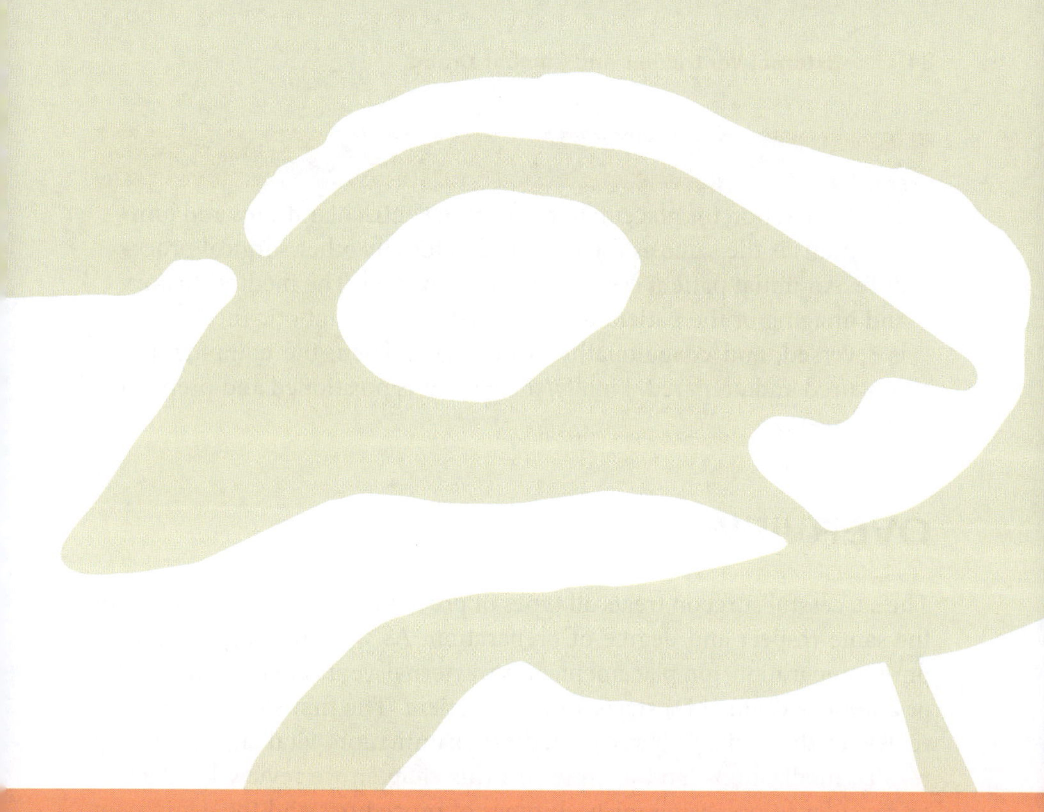

CHAPTER 3

Procedure Preparation

CHAPTER SUMMARY

The preparation for placement of external ventricular drains and lumbar drains is the same as the preparation for any other surgical procedure. An initial patient assessment is performed. The medical history and imaging of the patient are reviewed. Antithrombotic medication is reversed, and coagulopathy is managed. Then, the equipment is procured and prepared. Finally, the patient is positioned and prepped for surgery.

OVERVIEW

The successful surgeon treats all types of procedures, however minor, with the same respect and degree of preparation. As with any surgical procedure, preparation for placement of an external ventricular drain (EVD) or a lumbar drain (LD) starts with the patient. The first step is a detailed review of the patient's history, medical examination, vital signs, imaging results, medications, and allergies. In this chapter, we review key factors to consider in preparing for both types of procedures and the equipment needed for each.

INITIAL EVALUATION

Preliminary Survey

As is the case with any patient interaction, a preliminary assessment must be conducted not only of the patient undergoing placement of an EVD or an LD but also of the scene. First, what is the physical setting in which the drain is being placed? A chaotic emergency department presents a different challenge than the spacious and controlled environment of the operating room. A plan should be made for working among other care teams or taking priority over them and for moving around objects such as tables, monitors, and ventilators. The availability of staff should also be considered. Both EVD and LD placement are procedures that require at least two persons. A nurse, technician, advanced practice provider, or another physician can help position and monitor the patient while the procedure is ongoing or can help with handing off supplies.

Second, the condition of the patient is evaluated. The ABCs of basic life support (airway, breathing, circulation) must be assessed. Is the patient intubated? Or will intubation be needed before the drain is placed? Is the patient hypotensive or in cardiac arrest? If the patient is immediately moribund for nonneurologic reasons, this must be strongly considered when deciding whether a drain is appropriate. Is the patient combative or unable to follow commands? Innumerable examples of observations made by the neurosurgeon during this preliminary survey directly impact the care being given by the primary team.

History, Physical Examination, and Imaging

When preparing for an EVD placement, the surgeon should note whether the patient has had a previous cranial procedure. A prior craniotomy with plates or a craniectomy with mesh can alter the entrance site. Opening over mesh may not allow the catheter to pass through or may cause the catheter to be cut, damaged, or easily occluded. Pushing down on a bone flap may cause it to become dislodged. Reviewing the imaging facilitates detection of these features and enables measurement of bone thickness, distance to the foramen of Monro, and approach angles; identification of vessel or vascular abnormalities that may be at risk; and detection of any blood in the ventricles. An anterior communicating artery, an internal carotid artery terminus, or a basilar apex aneurysm can have a morphology that places the dome in the trajectory of the EVD. Anecdotal stories of piercing or cannulating an aneurysm or arteriovenous malformation are told among neurosurgeons, but case reports are rare. In an example from our experience, laterality of an EVD being placed had to be changed because bullet fragments were found in the trajectory. In patients with severe intraventricular hemorrhage, bilateral placement could be considered.[1] The skin must be examined to identify prior incisions or scars. Sites of breakdown, rash, and infection should be carefully noted, not only before drain placement but also after placement, because these sites may be associated with increased risk of a drain infection.

Before inserting an LD, the neurosurgeon must consider whether the patient has had previous lumbar surgery. A prior laminectomy may make access much easier, but it also removes the landmarks the neurosurgeon depends on. Spinal fusion may decrease or completely obliterate the interlaminar space because of bony growth. Scoliosis or morbid obesity should be a red flag that difficulty lies ahead. A lumboperitoneal shunt, intrathecal pump, or dorsal column stimulator can be damaged if it lies in the path of the drain. A review of the imaging will help confirm the types of previous surgery, lumbar stenosis, the quality of the interlaminar space, and the level of the conus medullaris, and it will help identify any existing hardware or devices. Evaluation of the patient should also focus on signs of infected or broken-down skin, surgical scars, and the girth of the lower back.

Antithrombotic Medication and Coagulopathy

One of the most important factors to consider is whether the patient takes any antithrombotic agent or has bleeding diathesis. A purposeful investigation of anticoagulant or antiplatelet medication use is necessary. If the patient or a family member cannot provide this information, it should be searched for in the chart. Meta-analyses have found a higher rate of hemorrhagic complications in patients who are given antiplatelet or anticoagulant therapy before EVD placement.[2,3] The evidence is not as strong for lumbar punctures or LDs, but anticoagulation may increase the risk compared to antiplatelet medication.[4]

Bleeding time, clotting time, prothrombin time, partial thromboplastin time, international normalized ratio (INR), and complete blood cell count have historically been used to assess coagulopathy, whether medication-induced or acquired. The drawbacks to these tests are that they do not provide complete pictures of hemostasis, platelet function, and the fibrinolytic pathway. Thromboelastography has evolved from its initial use in transplant surgery to its widespread application in several specialties. Thromboelastography, with or without platelet mapping, assesses the viscoelastic properties of blood as it forms a clot, giving a complete picture of the coagulation cascade, platelet function, and fibrinolytic system. We direct the readers to an excellent 2021 review on the subject by Shaydakov et al.[5] Thromboelastography has shown its value in cardiac, cirrhotic, and transplant surgery by reducing the need for transfusion products and decreasing thrombotic events; however, it has not yet shown promise in the trauma population.[6–8] We believe that thromboelastography is a more informative test than historical assays and recommend its routine use as part of the initial evaluation in all neurosurgery patients, including those who are to receive an EVD or LD.

Correcting medication or coagulopathy has not been studied as intensively in patients undergoing an EVD or LD placement as it has been in spontaneous intracranial hemorrhage (ICH) and cranial surgery. Therefore, we must apply this evidence to our focus. The offending medication should be discontinued or withheld in all cases, except for life-threatening pulmonary (eg, saddle) embolism or ICH secondary to venous thrombosis.

Knowledge of the specific actions of the different classes of agents can be aided by reviewing the coagulation cascade (Fig. 3.1). It has become the standard of care to urgently reverse coagulation in any patient with ICH

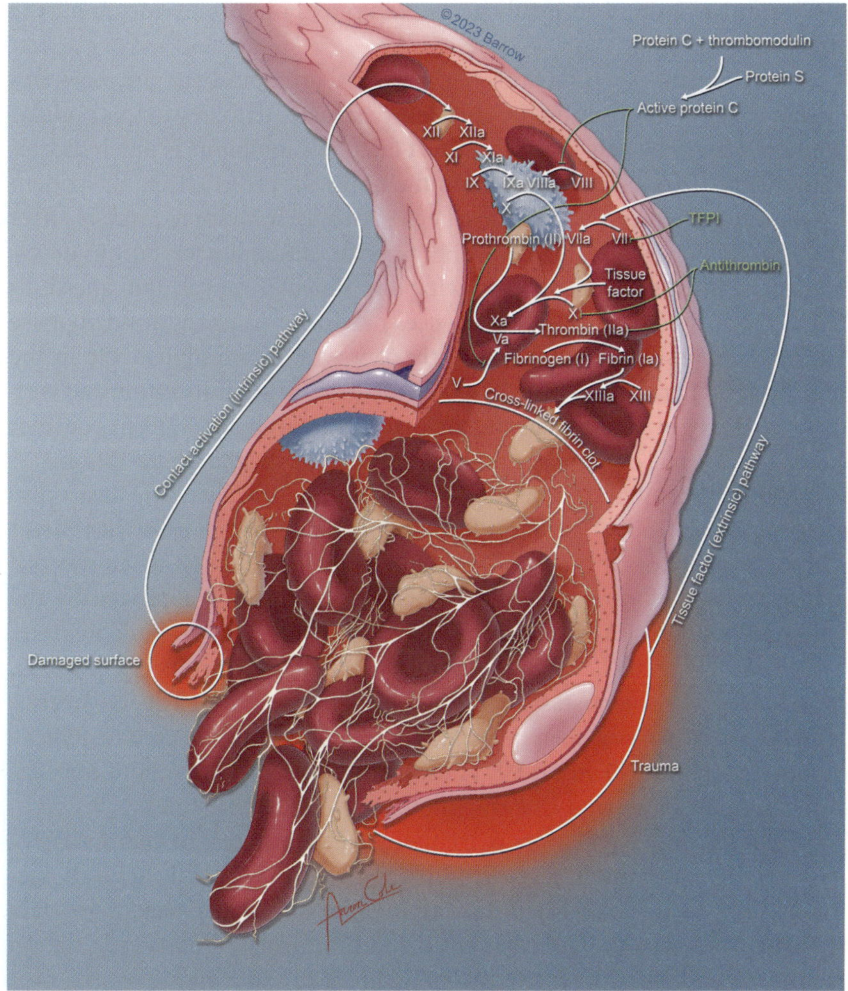

FIGURE 3.1. Artist's rendition of coagulation cascade. TFPI, tissue factor pathway inhibitor.

taking a vitamin K antagonist (VKA) such as warfarin.[9] The current recommendations suggest using a four-factor prothrombin complex concentrate (PCC) in addition to a 10-mg intravenous dose of vitamin K (PCC for immediate reversal, VKA for longer coverage). These recommendations are for patients with an INR >1.4 but must be weight-based, and the lowest dose is recommended for patients with an INR of 1.4 to 2.0. PCC is favored over fresh frozen plasma (FFP), given the increased risk of transfusion-associated complications.[9] A multicenter controlled trial has shown the benefit of PCC over FFP in reducing hemorrhage volume.[10] Recombinant factor VIIa is not recommended. INR should be checked frequently after the administration of reversal agents for up to 24 hours to document the effects of reversal.

Direct factor Xa inhibitors (eg, rivaroxaban, apixaban) are now frequently used. Consensus on the ideal test parameter to follow in this population is lacking. The half-life of the direct factor Xa inhibitors is much shorter than that of VKA and, depending on the timing of presentation, the patient may not require reversal.[9] PCC has been shown to have some reversal effect and is likely better tolerated than FFP.[9] Specific antibodies are now in development, with andexanet alfa showing prominent reversal, but questions remain regarding real-world experiences outside of company-funded phase 1 trials.[11,12] These antibodies will likely play a more prominent role in the near future. Therefore, in cases of recent medication administration and with the availability of reversal agents, the primary treatment team can consider either PCC or one of these antibodies, with FFP as the third-line option.[9]

Direct thrombin inhibitors (eg, dabigatran, bivalirudin, desirudin, argatroban, lepirudin) are used less frequently. As is the case with direct factor Xa inhibitors, timing to the last dose may be enough when reversal is not needed. Idarucizumab is a monoclonal antibody approved by the US Food and Drug Administration specifically for reversal of dabigatran. Three phase 1 trials[13–15] and a phase 3 trial[14] have shown its effectiveness in reversal, with hemostasis achieved with a low rate of adverse events. However, concern has been raised about the long time required to achieve hemostasis (about 11 hours).[16] Thus, in this patient population, idarucizumab remains a second-line treatment, with PCC third-line.[9]

Heparin anticoagulation is frequently encountered in neurosurgery patients. The administration of standard heparin indirectly inhibits factor Xa and factor IIa via antithrombin. Low-molecular-weight heparin (LMWH) binds to and activates antithrombin, which inhibits coagulation factors Xa and IIa. Current recommendations are to avoid reversing prophylactically dosed subcutaneous unfractionated heparin unless the activated partial thromboplastin time is significantly prolonged. In a patient with ICH receiving therapeutic heparin infusion, recommendations are to administer 1 mg of protamine for every 100 units of heparin given in the previous 2 to 3 hours, with a maximum single dose of 50 mg.[9] LMWHs (eg, enoxaparin) are less likely to be fully reversed by protamine. No large randomized controlled trials have been conducted, but current recommendations call for protamine to be given in a 1-mg dose per 1-mg enoxaparin (up to a maximum single dose of 50 mg) if enoxaparin was given within 8 hours, or a 0.5-mg dose per 1-mg enoxaparin if enoxaparin was given in the past 8 to 12 hours. If protamine is contraindicated, intravenous recombinant factor VIIa (90 μg/kg) is the second-line treatment.[9]

Pentasaccharides (eg, fondaparinux), which are not heparins, act by potentiating antithrombin's effect but do not respond to protamine. These drugs are less well-studied, but current recommendations are for activated PCC (20 IU/kg) as a first-line treatment and recombinant factor VIIa (90 µg/kg) as a second-line treatment.[9]

Plasminogen activators (PAs), also called thrombolytics, convert plasminogen to plasmin, which leads to the degradation of fibrinogen and fibrin. Fibrin-selective and fibrin-nonselective PAs are available. The selective PAs, such as recombinant tissue PA (rtPA) and tenecteplase, degrade only fibrin, whereas the nonselective PAs, such as urokinase and streptokinase, degrade both fibrin and fibrinogen (Fig. 3.2). ICH expansion after administration of rtPA is more likely to occur in patients with fibrinogen levels <150 mg/dL.[17] Cryoprecipitate is derived from FFP, and it contains fibrinogen (200 mg/U), factor VIII, fibronectin, factor XIII, and von Willebrand factor; 10 units is expected to raise levels by 70 mg/dL in a 70-kg patient.[17] The antifibrinolytics (eg, ε-aminocaproic acid, tranexamic acid) bind to plasminogen, which prevents its conversion to plasmin, thereby preventing fibrin degradation. The first-line treatment recommendation is to use 10 units of cryoprecipitate if thrombolytics have been given in the past 24 hours or the patient has a symptomatic hemorrhage. Fibrinogen levels should be rechecked after administration, and additional doses should be administered if levels are <150 mg/dL. Antifibrinolytic agents are used as a second-line treatment.[9] Antiplatelet agents target several receptors, including cyclooxygenase, adenosine diphosphate, phosphodiesterase, glycoprotein IIb/IIIa, thromboxane, and protease-activated receptor-1. Although a meta-analysis of retrospective studies failed to show a protective effect for platelet transfusion,[18] a randomized trial of patients receiving aspirin therapy who had ICH and were undergoing emergency craniotomy found that platelet transfusion significantly reduced the postoperative hemorrhage rate and volume, as well as the disability and mortality rates.[19] Desmopressin is an analog of vasopressin that promotes the endothelial release of factor VIII–von Willebrand complex. In a small study of 14 patients, desmopressin administration elicited a response in von Willebrand factor, with only two patients showing hematoma growth.[20] Thus, current recommendations are for platelet transfusion for patients undergoing a procedure who are receiving aspirin or adenosine diphosphate inhibitor therapy, with preoperative testing of platelet function, if possible.[9] This transfusion should be withheld when testing shows normal function or when patients are receiving glycoprotein IIb/IIIa inhibitors, which drastically inhibit receptors and reduce the likelihood that transfusion will be beneficial. Desmopressin can be administered in addition to a unit of platelets.[9] Table 3.1 summarizes the classes of antithrombotic medications and the first line of reversal.

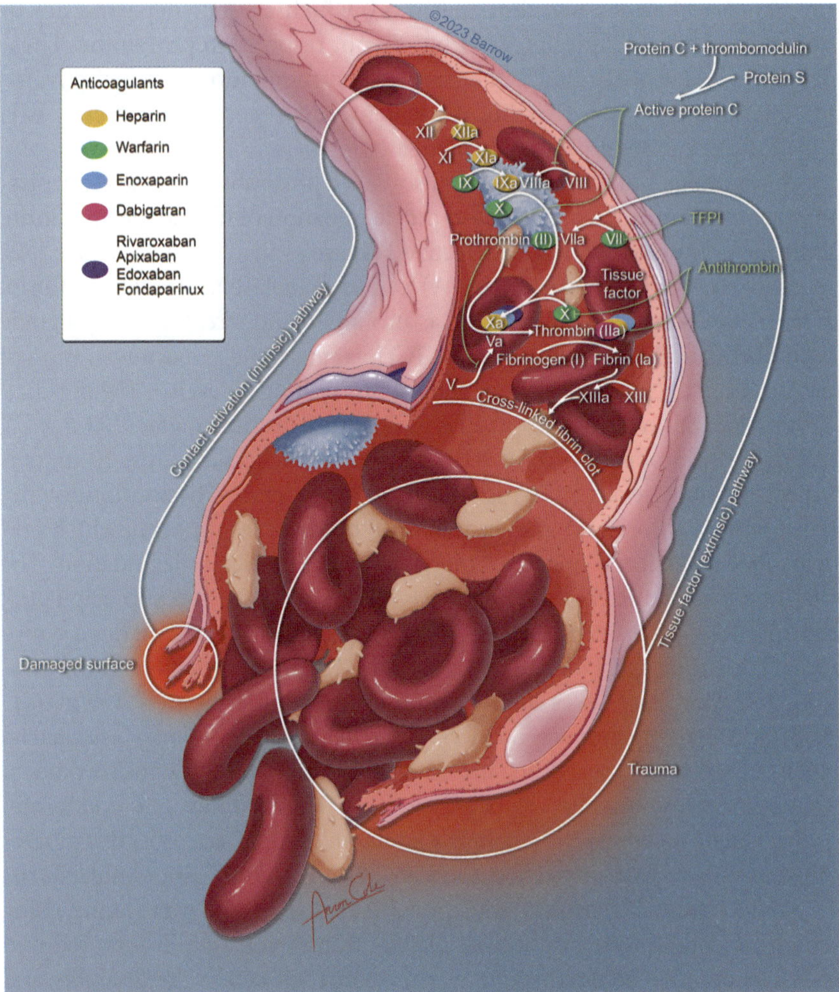

FIGURE 3.2. Review of coagulation cascade with the action point for each medication. TFPI, tissue factor pathway inhibitor.

In trauma patients, the CRASH-3 trial showed that tranexamic acid reduced the rate of head injury–related death when administered within 3 hours.[21,22] However, concerns have been raised about the effectiveness of tranexamic acid and the likelihood of thrombotic events with its use.[23]

The data are less robust in patients who have undergone lumbar punctures and LD placement. For example, the evidence on plasma transfusion for abnormal coagulation or platelet transfusion for thrombocytopenia is observational, at best.[24–26]

In summary, evaluating coagulopathy or the potential use of antithrombotic medication in a patient needing an EVD or LD requires standard

TABLE 3.1: ANTITHROMBOTIC AGENTS AND THEIR REVERSAL AGENTS

Antithrombotic Class	Primary Reversal Agent
Vitamin K antagonists	4-factor PCC, plus 10 mg IV vitamin K
Direct factor Xa inhibitors	PCC or andexanet alfa
Direct thrombin inhibitors	If not enough time has elapsed, use idarucizumab
Heparins	UFH: 1 mg protamine for every 100 U of heparin given in the previous 2 to 3 hours (50 mg maximum single dose)
	LMWH: 1 mg protamine per 1 mg LMWH administered if dosed within 8 hours (50 mg maximum single dose); 0.5 mg protamine per 1 mg LMWH if last dose was within 8 to 12 hours
Pentasaccharides	aPCC 20 IU/kg
Plasminogen activators	10 U cryoprecipitate; follow fibrinogen levels
Antiplatelets	1 U platelets if undergoing a procedure and concurrently on aspirin or ADP inhibitor therapy, with testing indicating platelet dysfunction

ADP, adenosine diphosphate; aPCC, activated prothrombin complex concentrate; IV, intravenous; LMWH, low-molecular-weight heparin; PCC, prothrombin complex concentrate; UFH, unfractionated heparin.

testing, with the addition of thromboelastography with or without platelet mapping. Medications should be withheld until after drain placement (the timing for restarting these medications is covered in Chap. 6, "Complication Management"). Correction of the effects of the coagulopathy or medication should be guided by existing recommendations, as well as the results of testing, evaluation of the patient's condition, and review of the dose of medication that the patient was taking.

PROCEDURE PREPARATION

Location and Staff

The hospital location where the drain is placed has been of interest lately; however, only retrospective data on the risks of the procedure by location exist at this point. One study showed the rate of complications to be significantly higher in patients with drains placed in the intensive care unit (ICU) compared with those placed in the operating room, but these patient populations were critically different in regard to prophylactic antibiotics, trauma, and intraventricular hemorrhage.[27] Other reports have been inconclusive, even when considering the assessment of infection.[28,29] Ultimately, the optimal hospital location for drain placement depends on the status of the patient and the inner working of the hospital. When a patient is in critical condition, time may not allow for an operating room or an ICU room to become available. Patients in an unstable condition may have added risk incurred by being transported from the ICU to the operating room. These factors should be taken into account to develop more definitive guidelines.

The extent of the experience of the surgeon placing the drain has been the subject of some discussion. Only retrospective data exist on this effect, which favors no difference in complications or success based on the years of training or the experience of the surgeon.[30-33] We believe that successful drain placement is like any other surgical procedure. The more often an EVD or LD placement is performed, the more likely placement is to be successful. This repetition is institution-dependent. A senior resident may place fewer drains than a pediatric neurosurgeon, but a junior resident may place more than a peripheral nerve specialist. Ultimately, surgeons should seek to improve their performance with any of the many modalities now in existence, including cadaveric courses, 3D-printed models, virtual simulators, and workshops.[34-36]

The growing need for neurocritical care coverage has led to a discussion about expanding the range of practitioners who can perform EVD placement. Retrospective data on the placement of EVDs and intracranial pressure monitors (ICPMs) by neurointensivists, general surgery residents, trauma surgeons, and advanced practice providers indicate rates of complications comparable to those of neurosurgeons.[37-41] We agree that the skills required to place EVDs and ICPMs with a low complication rate can be learned by a broad range of providers. However, we caution against equating comfort with the steps of the procedure to understanding the reasoning, anatomy, and management of drains and monitors. Placing an EVD or an ICPM without complications is not the same as placing a successful drain. Unlike any other critical care procedure (eg, arterial or venous line, endotracheal tube, thoracostomy tube), placement of EVDs and ICPMs requires the incorporation of detailed knowledge of the anatomy with an assessment of preprocedural imaging. These skills are taught over the course of neurosurgery residency and are only briefly reviewed in this book. Additionally, troubleshooting during drain or monitor placement and complication awareness are skills that are sharpened during cranial surgery experiences available only to neurosurgeons. We also caution against the luxury of drain placement without commitment to its long-term management, which is where the understanding of anatomy and physiology must be applied to produce a "successful" drain.

Finally, an argument can be made that unless providers can manage the complications that may arise from the procedure, they should not perform the procedure. For example, we once encountered major venous bleeding from a cortical vein that caused a large acute subdural hematoma requiring immediate decompressive craniotomy. Many reports have been made of rerupture of aneurysms after drain placement. In one meta-analysis, the average time to rerupture was within 1 hour of drain placement.[42] The management of these complications lies outside the scope of practice of neurointensivists and trauma surgeons, and their possibility should be considered with the placement of every drain. Therefore, if a patient needs an EVD, LD, or ICPM at an institution without immediate neurosurgery consultation and operative ability, we urge providers to carefully consider the risks and benefits of such placements. Instead, providers and patient representatives should engage in serious deliberation about transferring the patient to a facility with these capabilities.

Premedication

Before equipment needed for the drain is gathered, the appropriate medication for the procedure should be obtained. This process begins with identifying the medications necessary to provide the patient with comfort and pain relief.

When the procedure is being performed on a sedated or lethargic patient, the neurosurgeon must be prepared to have the patient intubated after the administration of medication. When the likelihood of airway compromise is high, it is safer to endotracheally intubate the patient prophylactically. Intubation is most frequently performed by emergency physicians, anesthesiologists, or intensivists.

First, proper intravenous access and pulse oximetry are ensured, with or without continuous end-tidal capnography. Then the patient is preoxygenated with 100% oxygen using a nonrebreather mask. The head of the bed is initially elevated to prevent pooling of secretions, and working suction is placed within reach. Some physicians may elect pretreatment to prevent an increase in blood pressure with laryngeal stimulation. Pretreatment typically involves the use of fentanyl or propofol, although care must be taken in hypotensive patients because such pretreatment may lower blood pressure and worsen cerebral perfusion.[43] The intubating physician then administers an induction agent, typically etomidate or ket-amine. Etomidate has mild hemodynamic effects, decreases cerebral blood flow, and decreases cerebral metabolic demand, but it does not provide an analgesic defect. Ketamine has analgesic effects and has minimal effect on blood pressure, but concerns have been raised about it elevating intra-cranial pressure.[43] The patient is then ventilated with a bag-valve-mask to ensure that oxygenation can be maintained in case intubation fails.

Next, a paralytic agent is given. Succinylcholine is the paralytic agent of choice because of its rapid onset and offset (60-90 seconds).[43] This depolarizing agent creates fasciculations, which has raised concern about increased ICP, although the degree to which this occurs is debatable. Rocuronium has been proposed as an alternative because it is nondepolar-izing and theoretically has a less pronounced effect on ICP. In a Cochrane Review, succinylcholine was reported to be superior to rocuronium for rapid sequence intubation,[44] but this finding has been questioned because it did not include patients with severe brain injury.[45]

Endotracheal intubation is then performed, and adequate placement is ensured with auscultation of lung sounds and end-tidal capnography. The endotracheal tube is secured. Postintubation, the patient is maintained on a combination of sedative and analgesic medications. This treatment is typically a combination of propofol and fentanyl drips or, if hypotension is a concern, a combination of midazolam and fentanyl or just a fentanyl drip by itself. A chest radiograph, depending on the ease of obtaining it, should be performed before or after tube placement to document the placement of the endotracheal tube.

For the more alert patient, we still recommend some form of continu-ous sedation and analgesia because an EVD procedure can be traumatizing. This can be accomplished with low-dose drips of fentanyl and midazolam. An LD is generally better tolerated, and the procedure can often be per-formed with a local anesthetic alone.

Vital signs are monitored frequently, especially after the administration of medication. Continuous monitoring of arterial blood pressure, capnography, and pulse oximetry should be conducted. A final consideration of necessary premedication is prophylactic intravenous antibiotics. Such premedication has been the subject of randomized trials as well as systematic reviews, and we review it in-depth in our discussion of catheters in this chapter.

Equipment

The last step of preparation is to ensure that all the necessary equipment to perform an EVD or LD placement has been gathered and placed at the beside before beginning the procedure. At the University of Rochester, the practice was once to obtain each item of equipment piece by piece, but it soon became clear that doing so hampered the surgeon's ability to perform the procedure quickly. Instead, a prefilled "ready bag" is now prepared for each type of drain. The ready bag is a large duffle bag that contains all the necessary equipment to complete the procedure (Fig. 3.3). Having a ready bag prepared in advance for EVDs and LDs allows the hospital to restock and account for parts easily. Time trials revealed a significant reduction in the time needed to start the procedure, saving an average of 13 minutes per procedure ($p < 0.001$).[46] The prefilled bag can be modified to also include ICPM components. These ready bags can be strategically placed in the ICU, the emergency department, operating rooms, or even other hospitals within the overall healthcare system, where they can be maintained by the material managers of each unit. The bags should be checked daily and tagged when restocked, with the tag placed within the bag when broken after equipment is used. At our institution, we have at least three EVD and three LD bags operational at any time. Tables 3.2 and 3.3 list the contents of the equipment in the EVD ready bag (Fig. 3.4) and the LD ready bag (Fig. 3.5), respectively.

Drain-related infections can be devastating for patients, and their prevention is paramount. Prophylactic antibiotics and the type of catheter that is used are of particular importance and have been subject to considerable investigation, including multiple randomized controlled trials and systematic reviews with meta-analyses.[47–54] The most recent meta-analysis reported in 2020 by Sheppard et al[54] included over 19 studies with 5242 patients. Their minimum definition for drain-related infection included a positive cerebrospinal fluid (CSF) culture result, a positive blood culture result, or CSF leukocytosis. Across the 19 studies, these authors found an average infection rate of 23.1% without any intervention. The addition of antibiotic prophylaxis for less than 24 hours reduced the infection rate to 11.7%. Adding an antibiotic-coated catheter to short-term antibiotic prophylaxis reduced the infection rate even further to 4.9%. This rate was similar to that for long-term antibiotic prophylaxis without antibiotic-coated catheters (4.7%). The most profound reduction was noted with a combination of long-term antibiotic prophylaxis with antibiotic-coated catheters, which reduced the average infection rate to 0.8%. In the financial analysis, antibiotic-coated catheters with long-term coverage produced the highest savings compared to the costs for patients with no intervention or with short-term antibiotic treatment, which saved slightly less. We believe that patients undergoing the placement of EVDs and LDs should be treated the same as patients undergoing any other surgical procedure. A prophylactic

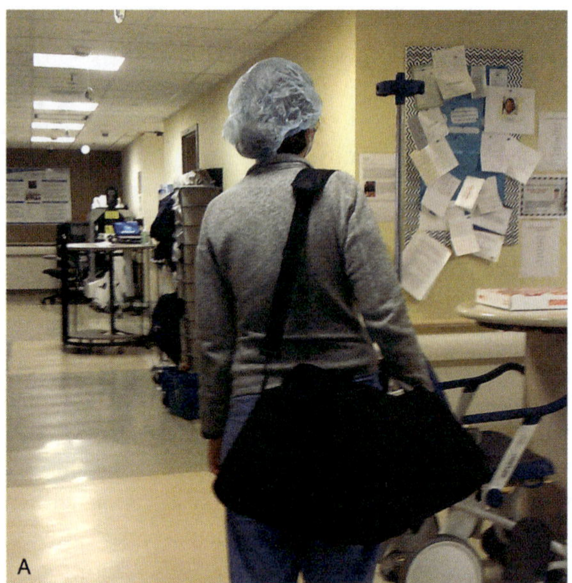

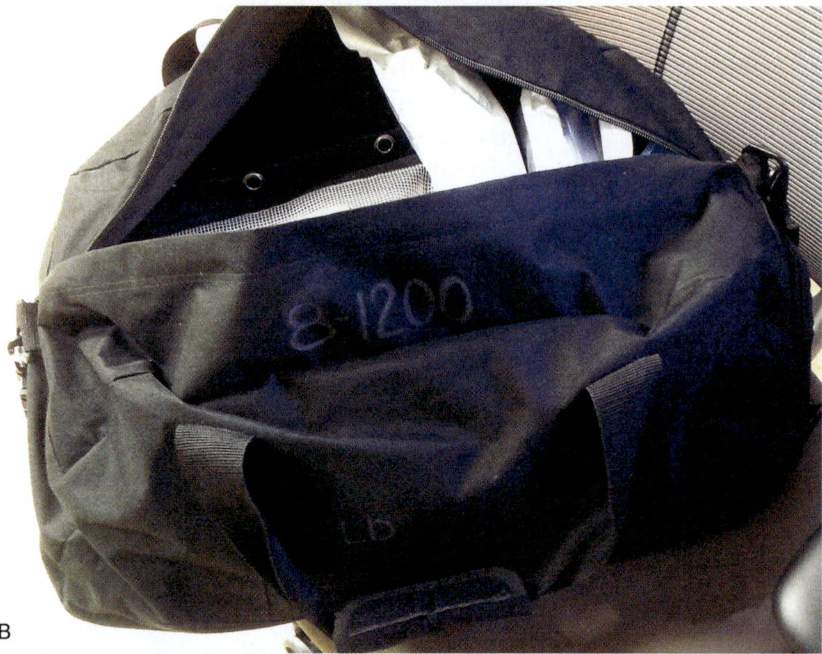

FIGURE 3.3. External ventricular drain (EVD) equipment bag. **A.** An EVD ready bag should contain all the equipment necessary for the drain and should be easy to carry. **B.** The bag should be clearly marked with the type of drain it contains and its proper location in the hospital, then tied with a marker to signify the drain has been restocked.

TABLE 3.2: THE EXTERNAL VENTRICULAR DRAIN READY BAG USED BY THE DEPARTMENT OF NEUROSURGERY AT THE UNIVERSITY OF ROCHESTER

Contents

- Cranial access kit
- Antibiotic-impregnated catheter
- CSF collection chamber
- CSF collection chamber transducer
- Transducer cable
- Sterile forceps
- Sterile needle driver
- Sterile scissors
- 4-0 Silk suture, without needle
- 2-0 Nylon sutures (4 needed)
- 1 Pack sterile blue towels
- 2 Chlorhexidine scrub sticks or 1 bottle povidone-iodine
- Chlorhexidine scrub sponge
- 1 Bottle sterile normal saline
- Assortment of sterile gloves in various sizes
- Sterile marking pens
- Scrub hats
- Face shields
- 2 Sterile gowns
- BioPatch disc
- Sterile half drape
- Sterile drain cover gauze
- Perforated tape
- Sterile normal saline syringes
- Sterile red caps

CSF, cerebrospinal fluid.

course of antibiotics, based on the institutional microbiome, should be administered and continued for no longer than 24 hours. In all EVD cases, an antibiotic-coated catheter should be used (Fig. 3.6). Antibiotic-coated LD catheters are not as readily accessible and would be a meaningful item for biomedical producers to distribute.

BioPatch (Ethicon; Johnson & Johnson) and chlorhexidine-based sponges have been shown to reduce bacterial colonization in epidural catheter exit sites and central venous catheters.[55–57] Thus, at the University of Rochester, their use is part of the procedures for both EVD and LD placement (Fig. 3.7). Although the supportive data are not as strong for Ioban (3M Co.), it is also the policy to use Ioban as the occlusive dressing for patients undergoing an LD placement (Fig. 3.8).

TABLE 3.3: THE LUMBAR DRAIN READY BAG USED BY THE DEPARTMENT OF NEUROSURGERY AT THE UNIVERSITY OF ROCHESTER

Contents
• Lumbar puncture kit
• Lumbar catheters (open tip and closed tip)
• CSF collection chamber
• CSF collection chamber transducer
• Transducer cable
• Sterile forceps
• Sterile needle driver
• Sterile scissors
• 4-0 Silk suture, without needle
• 4-0 Nylon sutures (2 needed)
• 1 Pack sterile blue towels
• 1 Bottle betadine or 2 chlorhexidine scrub sticks
• 1 Bottle sterile normal saline
• Assortment of sterile gloves in various sizes
• Sterile marking pens
• Scrub hats
• Face shields
• 2 Sterile gowns
• Ioban (medium size)
• BioPatch disc
• Sterile half drape
• Sterile normal saline syringes
• Sterile red caps

CSF, cerebrospinal fluid.

A final important consideration is whether an adjunct should be used to improve the accuracy of the drain placement. For an LD, imaging-guided access would require a separate consultation with interventional radiology in most hospitals. Thus, whether to use imaging guidance must be considered ahead of time when possible, and it will likely not be available in emergency situations. For EVDs, the adjunct that has received the most attention is stereotactic neuronavigation. AlAzri et al[58] conducted a retrospective study and found that the use of navigation (not surprisingly) significantly improved the accuracy of placement and significantly reduced the number of passes necessary to complete the procedure ($p < 0.02$). In a prospective single-arm trial of neuronavigation in the ICU that enrolled 35 patients, Mahan et al[59] found that navigation significantly

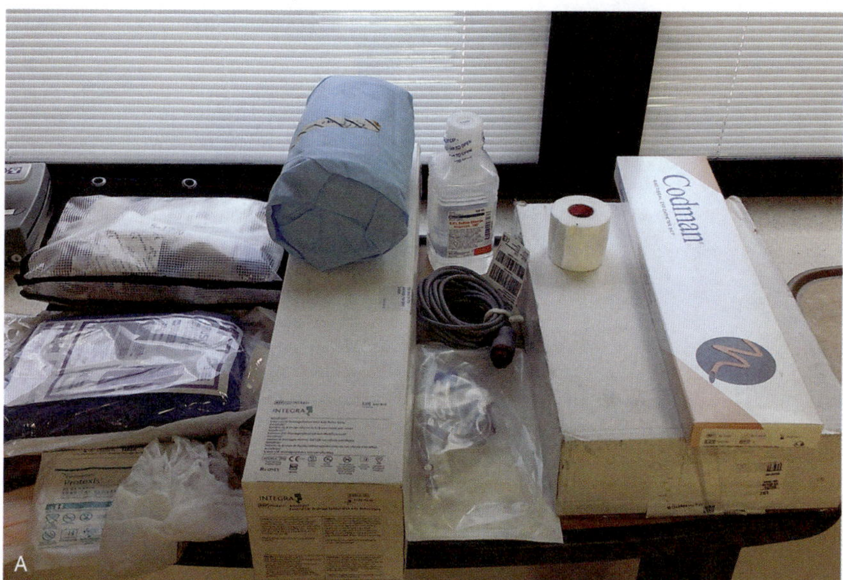

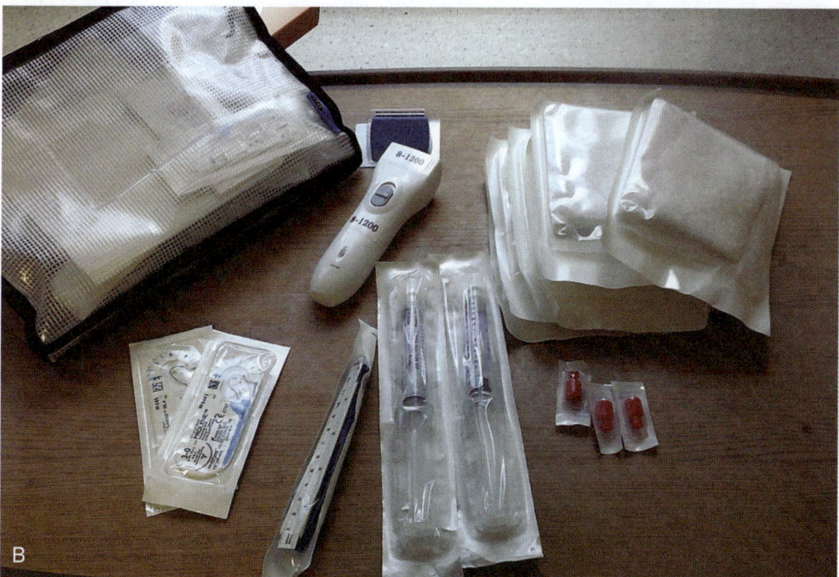

FIGURE 3.4. Contents of an external ventricular drain (EVD) equipment bag. **A.** An EVD ready bag should include the catheter, collection chamber, cranial access kit, and sterilizing solutions (please refer to Table 3.2 for a full list of contents). **B.** A resealable pouch, which is stocked with small, loose items, such as flushes, sterile caps, and markers, can be placed in the ready bag.

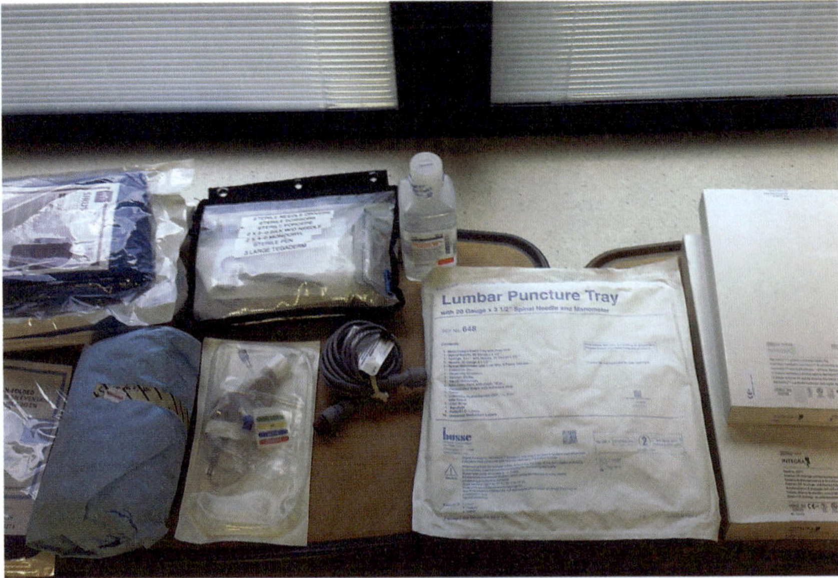

FIGURE 3.5. Lumbar drain (LD) equipment bag contents. In addition to the LD catheter box, the contents of the LD ready bag may include a lumbar puncture tray, which also contains a manometer for measuring opening pressure, the collection chamber, and the sterilizing solution (please refer to Table 3.3 for a full list of contents).

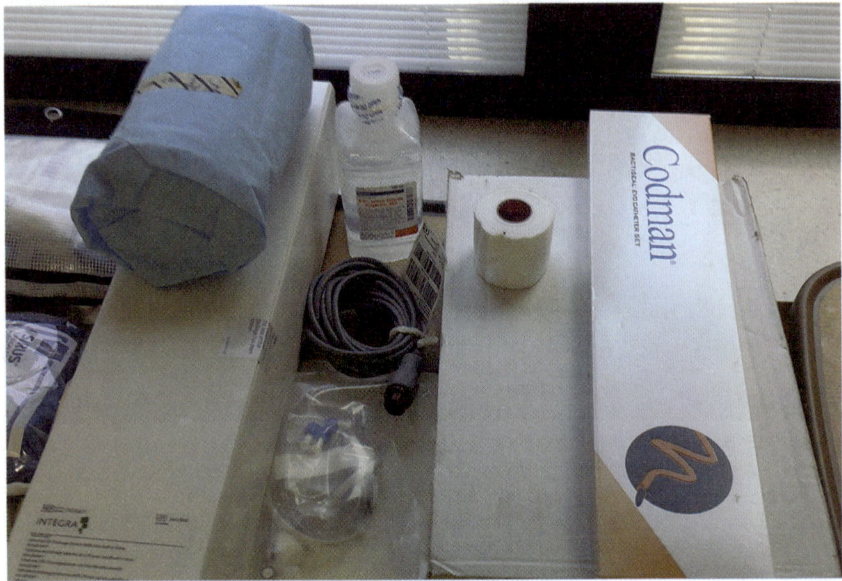

FIGURE 3.6. An antibiotic-impregnated catheter should be part of any external ventricular drain kit. Unfortunately, antibiotic-impregnated catheters do not currently exist for lumbar drains.

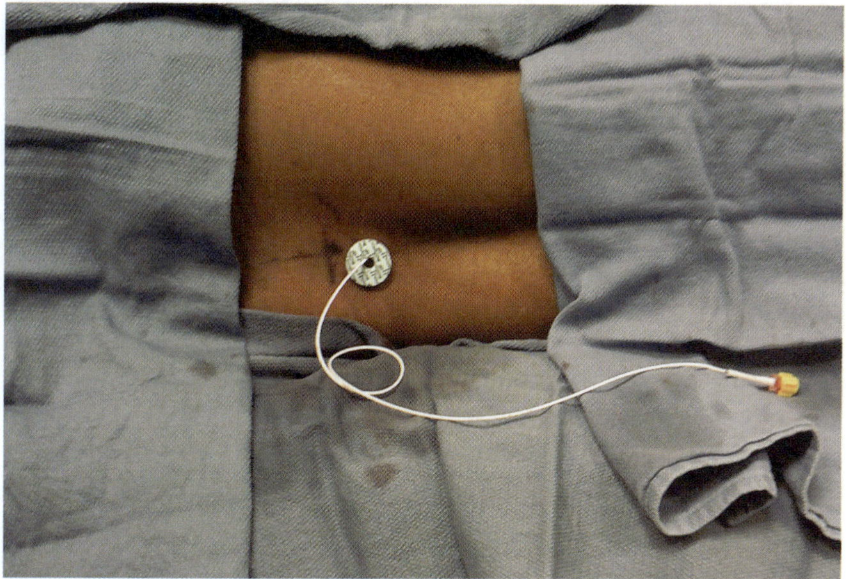

FIGURE 3.7. A BioPatch should be part of the kit for both the external ventricular drain and the lumbar drain. The BioPatch can be placed around the drain at its skin exit site.

improved accuracy, with only one tract hemorrhage identified ($p < 0.001$). The addition of neuronavigation added approximately 36 minutes of procedure time.

In some countries, most EVDs are placed in the operating room, which facilitates the use of real-time ultrasound through the two burr holes to place the catheter.[60] In a retrospective study comparing freehand neuronavigation and ultrasound-guided placement of the ventricular catheters of shunts, Wilson et al[61] found that neuronavigation and ultrasound both significantly improved accuracy ($p < 0.001$). Some authors have reported trialing newer technologies such as smartphone-based navigation and mixed-reality holographic wearable navigation.[62,63] Others have described using the iGuide navigational guidance system (Siemens AG) in the angiography suite to place EVDs accurately.[64]

In many countries, especially those in Europe, accuracy has been improved by adopting an implant-based approach rather than navigation-based methods. This approach involves using a screw-in bolt after making the craniotomy hole, which theoretically maintains an orthogonal trajectory better than a freehand pass. In the largest review of the bolt technique to date, Roach et al[65] conducted a retrospective analysis of 579 patients that found the accuracy to be similar to that of tunneled EVD placements.

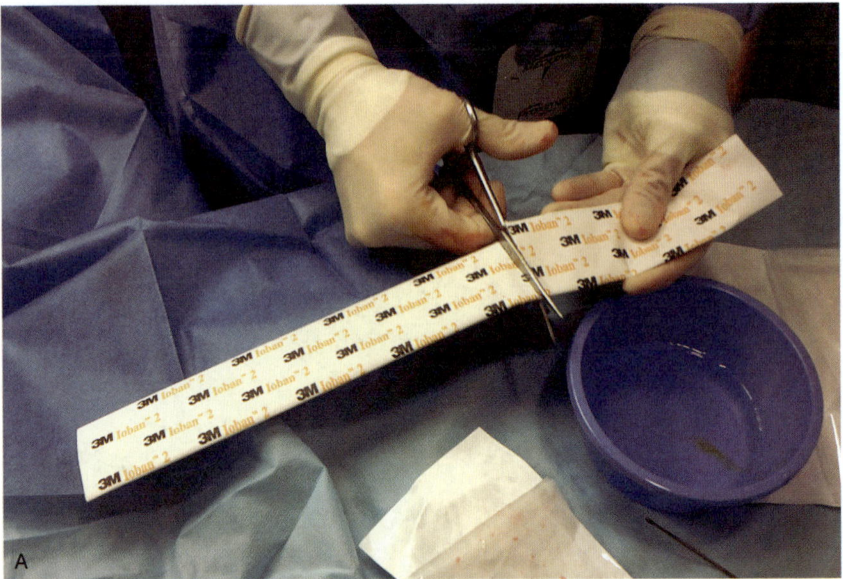

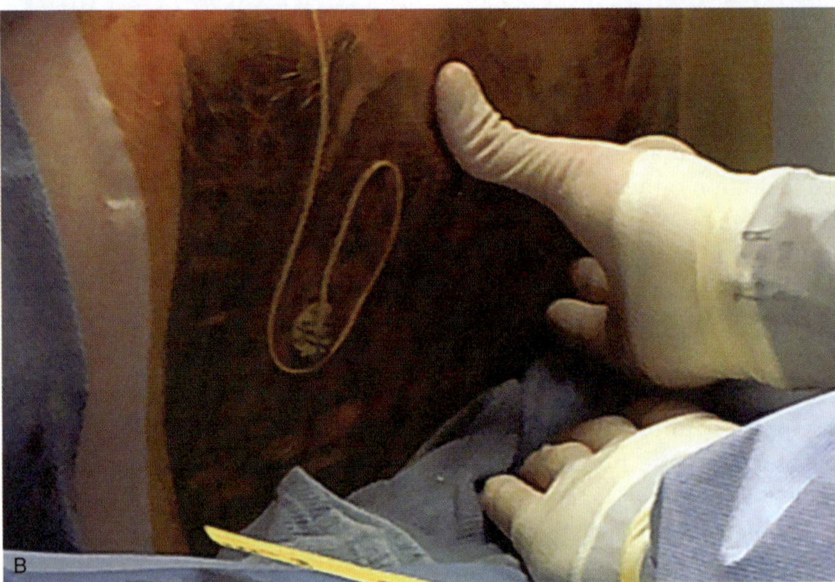

FIGURE 3.8. The kits for the external ventricular drain and the lumbar drain (LD) also include medium sheets of Ioban **(A)** for use as the occlusive dressing for the LD **(B)**.

Prospective studies of this modification of the EVD placement technique should be conducted before any recommendation can be made for its widespread adoption.

The utility of placing most EVDs in the operating room is debatable and depends on the institution or even the country. With the increase of technological investments in ICUs and EDs and the advancements in frameless neuronavigation, one can foresee these systems ultimately being made available in these locations. Neurosurgeons have become quite facile with this technology, even to the point of being able to register a patient in minutes, which makes the use of EVDs possible even in emergency situations.

ABBREVIATIONS

CSF, cerebrospinal fluid

EVD, external ventricular drain

FFP, fresh frozen plasma

ICH, intracranial hemorrhage

ICPM, intracranial pressure monitor

ICU, intensive care unit

INR, international normalized ratio

LD, lumbar drain

LMWH, low-molecular-weight heparin

PA, plasminogen activator

PCC, prothrombin complex concentrate

rtPA, recombinant tissue plasminogen activator

VKA, vitamin K antagonist

REFERENCES

1. Hinson HE, Melnychuk E, Muschelli J, Hanley DF, Awad IA, Ziai WC. Drainage efficiency with dual versus single catheters in severe intraventricular hemorrhage. *Neurocrit Care*. 2012;16(3):399-405. doi:10.1007/s12028-011-9569-9.
2. Zhu X. The hemorrhage risk of prophylactic external ventricular drain insertion in aneurysmal subarachnoid hemorrhage patients requiring endovascular aneurysm treatment: a systematic review and meta-analysis. *J Neurosurg Sci*. 2017;61(1):53-63. doi:10.23736/S0390-5616.16.03244-6.
3. Cagnazzo F, Di Carlo DT, Petrella G, Perrini P. Ventriculostomy-related hemorrhage in patients on antiplatelet therapy for endovascular treatment of acutely ruptured intracranial aneurysms: a meta-analysis. *Neurosurg Rev*. 2020;43(2):397-406. doi:10.1007/s10143-018-0999-0.
4. Domingues R, Bruniera G, Brunale F, Mangueira C, Senne C. Lumbar puncture in patients using anticoagulants and antiplatelet agents. *Arq Neuropsiquiatr*. 2016;74(8):679-686. doi:10.1590/0004-282X20160098.

5. Shaydakov ME, Sigmon DF, Blebea J. Thromboelastography. In: *StatPearls*. Treasure Island, FL: StatPearls Publishing; 2022. https://pubmed.ncbi.nlm.nih.gov/30725746/.

6. Deppe AC, Weber C, Zimmermann J, et al. Point-of-care thromboelastography/thromboelastometry-based coagulation management in cardiac surgery: a meta-analysis of 8332 patients. *J Surg Res.* 2016;203(2):424-433. doi:10.1016/j.jss.2016.03.008.

7. Kovalic AJ, Khan MA, Malaver D, et al. Thromboelastography versus standard coagulation testing in the assessment and reversal of coagulopathy among cirrhotics: a systematic review and meta-analysis. *Eur J Gastroenterol Hepatol.* 2020;32(3):291-302. doi:10.1097/MEG.0000000000001588.

8. Hunt H, Stanworth S, Curry N, et al. Thromboelastography (TEG) and rotational thromboelastometry (ROTEM) for trauma induced coagulopathy in adult trauma patients with bleeding. *Cochrane Database Syst Rev.* 2015;(2):CD010438. doi:10.1002/14651858. CD010438.pub2.

9. Frontera JA, Lewin JJ 3rd, Rabinstein AA, et al. Guideline for reversal of antithrombotics in intracranial hemorrhage: a statement for healthcare professionals from the Neurocritical Care Society and Society of Critical Care Medicine. *Neurocrit Care.* 2016;24(1):6-46. doi:10.1007/s12028-015-0222-x.

10. Steiner T, Poli S, Griebe M, et al. Fresh frozen plasma versus prothrombin complex concentrate in patients with intracranial haemorrhage related to vitamin K antagonists (INCH): a randomised trial. *Lancet Neurol.* 2016;15(6):566-573. doi:10.1016/ S1474-4422(16)00110-1.

11. Siegal DM, Curnutte JT, Connolly SJ, et al. Andexanet alfa for the reversal of factor Xa inhibitor activity. *N Engl J Med.* 2015;373(25):2413-2424. doi:10.1056/NEJMoa1510991.

12. Brown CS, Scott RA, Sridharan M, Rabinstein AA. Real-world utilization of andexanet alfa. *Am J Emerg Med.* 2020;38(4):810-814. doi:10.1016/j.ajem.2019.12.008.

13. Glund S, Stangier J, van Ryn J, et al. Effect of age and renal function on idarucizumab pharmacokinetics and idarucizumab-mediated reversal of dabigatran anticoagulant activity in a randomized, double-blind, crossover Phase Ib study. *Clin Pharmacokinet.* 2017;56(1):41-54. doi:10.1007/s40262-016-0417-0.

14. Pollack CV Jr, Reilly PA, Eikelboom J, et al. Idarucizumab for dabigatran reversal. *N Engl J Med.* 2015;373(6):511-520. doi:10.1056/NEJMoa1502000.

15. Glund S, Moschetti V, Norris S, et al. A randomised study in healthy volunteers to investigate the safety, tolerability and pharmacokinetics of idarucizumab, a specific antidote to dabigatran. *Thromb Haemost.* 2015;113(5):943-951. doi:10.1160/TH14-12-1080.

16. Gottlieb M, Khishfe B. Idarucizumab for the reversal of dabigatran. *Ann Emerg Med.* 2017;69(5):554-558. doi:10.1016/j.annemergmed.2016.11.025.

17. Yaghi S, Boehme AK, Dibu J, et al. Treatment and outcome of thrombolysis-related hemorrhage: a multicenter retrospective study. *JAMA Neurol.* 2015;72(12):1451-1457. doi:10.1001/jamaneurol.2015.2371.

18. Leong LB, David TK. Is platelet transfusion effective in patients taking antiplatelet agents who suffer an intracranial hemorrhage? *J Emerg Med.* 2015;49(4):561-572. doi:10.1016/j.jemermed.2015.02.023.

19. Li X, Sun Z, Zhao W, et al. Effect of acetylsalicylic acid usage and platelet transfusion on postoperative hemorrhage and activities of daily living in patients with acute intracerebral hemorrhage. *J Neurosurg.* 2013;118(1):94-103. doi:10.3171/2012.9.JNS112286.

20. Naidech AM, Maas MB, Levasseur-Franklin KE, et al. Desmopressin improves platelet activity in acute intracerebral hemorrhage. *Stroke.* 2014;45(8):2451-2453. doi:10.1161/ STROKEAHA.114.006061.

21. CRASH-3 Trial Collaborators. Effects of tranexamic acid on death, disability, vascular occlusive events and other morbidities in patients with acute traumatic brain injury (CRASH-3): a randomised, placebo-controlled trial. *Lancet.* 2019;394(10210):1713-1723. doi:10.1016/S0140-6736(19)32233-0.

22. Roberts I, Shakur-Still H, Aeron-Thomas A, et al. Tranexamic acid to reduce head injury death in people with traumatic brain injury: the CRASH-3 international RCT. *Health Technol Assess.* 2021;25(26):1-76. doi:10.3310/hta25260.

23. Chakroun-Walha O, Samet A, Jerbi M, et al. Benefits of the tranexamic acid in head trauma with no extracranial bleeding: a prospective follow-up of 180 patients. *Eur J Trauma Emerg Surg.* 2019;45(4):719-726. doi:10.1007/s00068-018-0974-z.

24. Estcourt LJ, Desborough MJ, Doree C, Hopewell S, Stanworth SJ. Plasma transfusions prior to lumbar punctures and epidural catheters for people with abnormal coagulation. *Cochrane Database Syst Rev.* 2017;9:CD012497. doi:10.1002/14651858.CD012497.pub2.

25. Estcourt LJ, Malouf R, Hopewell S, Doree C, Van Veen J. Use of platelet transfusions prior to lumbar punctures or epidural anaesthesia for the prevention of complications in people with thrombocytopenia. *Cochrane Database Syst Rev.* 2018;4:CD011980. doi:10.1002/14651858.CD011980.pub3.

26. Choi S, Brull R. Neuraxial techniques in obstetric and non-obstetric patients with common bleeding diatheses. *Anesth Analg.* 2009;109(2):648-660. doi:10.1213/ane.0b013e3181ac13d1.

27. Foreman PM, Hendrix P, Griessenauer CJ, Schmalz PG, Harrigan MR. External ventricular drain placement in the intensive care unit versus operating room: evaluation of complications and accuracy. *Clin Neurol Neurosurg.* 2015;128:94-100. doi:10.1016/j.clineuro.2014.09.026.

28. Kohli G, Singh R, Herschman Y, Mammis A. Infection incidence associated with external ventriculostomy placement: a comparison of outcomes in the emergency department, intensive care unit, and operating room. *World Neurosurg.* 2018;110:e135-e140. doi:10.1016/j.wneu.2017.10.129.

29. Dawod G, Henkel N, Karim N, et al. Does the setting of external ventricular drain placement affect morbidity? A systematic literature review comparing intensive care unit versus operating room procedures. *World Neurosurg.* 2020;140:131-141. doi:10.1016/j.wneu.2020.04.215.

30. Kakarla UK, Kim LJ, Chang SW, Theodore N, Spetzler RF. Safety and accuracy of bedside external ventricular drain placement. *Neurosurgery.* 2008;63(1 Suppl 1):ONS162-6; discussion ONS166-7. doi:10.1227/01.neu.0000335031.23521.d0.

31. Lee KS, Zhang JJY, Bolem N, et al. Freehand insertion of external ventricular drainage catheter: evaluation of accuracy in a single center. *Asian J Neurosurg.* 2020;15(1):45-50. doi:10.4103/ajns.AJNS_292_19.

32. Woernle CM, Burkhardt JK, Bellut D, Krayenbuehl N, Bertalanffy H. Do iatrogenic factors bias the placement of external ventricular catheters? A single institute experience and review of the literature. *Neurol Med Chir (Tokyo).* 2011;51(3):180-186. doi:10.2176/nmc.51.180.

33. Yuen J, Selbi W, Muquit S, Berei T. Complication rates of external ventricular drain insertion by surgeons of different experience. *Ann R Coll Surg Engl.* 2018;100(3):221-225. doi:10.1308/rcsann.2017.0221.

34. Bow H, He L, Raees MA, Pruthi S, Chitale R. Development and implementation of an inexpensive, easily producible, time efficient external ventricular drain simulator

using 3-dimensional printing and image registration. *Oper Neurosurg (Hagerstown).* 2019;16(4):496-502. doi:10.1093/ons/opy142.

35. Schirmer CM, Elder JB, Roitberg B, Lobel DA. Virtual reality-based simulation training for ventriculostomy: an evidence-based approach. *Neurosurgery.* 2013;73(Suppl 1): 66-73. doi:10.1227/NEU.0000000000000074.

36. Dasgupta D, D'Antona L, Aimone Cat D, et al. Simulation workshops as an adjunct to perioperative care bundles in the management of external ventricular drains: improving surgical technique and reducing infection. *J Neurosurg.* 2018:1-5. doi:10.3171/2018. 5.JNS172881.

37. Sadaka F, Kasal J, Lakshmanan R, Palagiri A. Placement of intracranial pressure monitors by neurointensivists: case series and a systematic review. *Brain Inj.* 2013;27(5):600-604. doi:10.3109/02699052.2013.772238.

38. Ekeh AP, Ilyas S, Saxe JM, et al. Successful placement of intracranial pressure monitors by trauma surgeons. *J Trauma Acute Care Surg.* 2014;76(2):286-290; discussion 290-291. doi:10.1097/TA.0000000000000092.

39. Enriquez-Marulanda A, Ascanio LC, Salem MM, et al. Accuracy and safety of external ventricular drain placement by physician assistants and nurse practitioners in aneurysmal acute subarachnoid hemorrhage. *Neurocrit Care.* 2018;29(3):435-442. doi:10.1007/s12028-018-0556-2.

40. Ellens NR, Fischer DL, Meldau JE, Schroeder BA, Patra SE. External ventricular drain placement accuracy and safety when done by midlevel practitioners. *Neurosurgery.* 2019;84(1):235-241. doi:10.1093/neuros/nyy090.

41. Young PJ, Bowling WM. Midlevel practitioners can safely place intracranial pressure monitors. *J Trauma Acute Care Surg.* 2012;73(2):431-434. doi:10.1097/TA. 0b013e318262437b.

42. Cagnazzo F, Gambacciani C, Morganti R, Perrini P. Aneurysm rebleeding after placement of external ventricular drainage: a systematic review and meta-analysis. *Acta Neurochir (Wien).* 2017;159(4):695-704. doi:10.1007/s00701-017-3124-1.

43. Kramer N, Lebowitz D, Walsh M, Ganti L. Rapid sequence intubation in traumatic brain-injured adults. *Cureus.* 2018;10(4):e2530. doi:10.7759/cureus.2530.

44. Tran DT, Newton EK, Mount VA, Lee JS, Wells GA, Perry JJ. Rocuronium versus succinylcholine for rapid sequence induction intubation. *Cochrane Database Syst Rev.* 2015;(10):CD002788. doi:10.1002/14651858.CD002788.pub3.

45. Patanwala AE, Erstad BL, Roe DJ, Sakles JC. Succinylcholine is associated with increased mortality when used for rapid sequence intubation of severely brain injured patients in the emergency department. *Pharmacotherapy.* 2016;36(1):57-63. doi:10.1002/phar. 1683.

46. Rahmani R, Houk C, Gargan C, Paulzak A, Fodness J, Roberts D. Minimizing door to treatment time: creating a "go bag" for external ventricular drain placement. *World J Surg Surgical Res.* 2020;3:1200.

47. Cui Z, Wang B, Zhong Z, et al. Impact of antibiotic- and silver-impregnated external ventricular drains on the risk of infections: a systematic review and meta-analysis. *Am J Infect Control.* 2015;43(7):e23-e32. doi:10.1016/j.ajic.2015.03.015.

48. Sonabend AM, Korenfeld Y, Crisman C, Badjatia N, Mayer SA, Connolly ES Jr. Prevention of ventriculostomy-related infections with prophylactic antibiotics and antibiotic-coated external ventricular drains: a systematic review. *Neurosurgery.* 2011;68(4): 996-1005. doi:10.1227/NEU.0b013e3182096d84.

49. Zabramski JM, Whiting D, Darouiche RO, et al. Efficacy of antimicrobial-impregnated external ventricular drain catheters: a prospective, randomized, controlled trial. *J Neurosurg.* 2003;98(4):725-730. doi:10.3171/jns.2003.98.4.0725.

50. Wong GK, Poon WS, Lyon D, Wai S. Cefepime vs. Ampicillin/Sulbactam and Aztreonam as antibiotic prophylaxis in neurosurgical patients with external ventricular drain: result of a prospective randomized controlled clinical trial. *J Clin Pharm Ther.* 2006;31(3):231-235. doi:10.1111/j.1365-2710.2006.00729.x.

51. Wang X, Dong Y, Qi XQ, Li YM, Huang CG, Hou LJ. Clinical review: efficacy of antimicrobial-impregnated catheters in external ventricular drainage: a systematic review and meta-analysis. *Crit Care.* 2013;17(4):234. doi:10.1186/cc12608.

52. Konstantelias AA, Vardakas KZ, Polyzos KA, Tansarli GS, Falagas ME. Antimicrobial-impregnated and -coated shunt catheters for prevention of infections in patients with hydrocephalus: a systematic review and meta-analysis. *J Neurosurg.* 2015;122(5): 1096-112. doi:10.3171/2014.12.JNS14908.

53. Pople I, Poon W, Assaker R, et al. Comparison of infection rate with the use of antibiotic-impregnated vs standard extraventricular drainage devices: a prospective, randomized controlled trial. *Neurosurgery.* 2012;71(1):6-13. doi:10.1227/NEU.0b013e3182544e31.

54. Sheppard JP, Ong V, Lagman C, et al. Systemic antimicrobial prophylaxis and antimicrobial-coated external ventricular drain catheters for preventing ventriculostomy-related infections: a meta-analysis of 5242 cases. *Neurosurgery.* 2020;86(1):19-29. doi:10.1093/neuros/nyy522.

55. Mann TJ, Orlikowski CE, Gurrin LC, Keil AD. The effect of the biopatch, a chlorhexidine impregnated dressing, on bacterial colonization of epidural catheter exit sites. *Anaesth Intensive Care.* 2001;29(6):600-603. doi:10.1177/0310057X0102900606.

56. Levy I, Katz J, Solter E, et al. Chlorhexidine-impregnated dressing for prevention of colonization of central venous catheters in infants and children: a randomized controlled study. *Pediatr Infect Dis J.* 2005;24(8):676-679. doi:10.1097/01.inf.0000172934.98865.14.

57. Timsit JF, Schwebel C, Bouadma L, et al. Chlorhexidine-impregnated sponges and less frequent dressing changes for prevention of catheter-related infections in critically ill adults: a randomized controlled trial. *JAMA.* 2009;301(12):1231-1241. doi:10.1001/jama.2009.376.

58. AlAzri A, Mok K, Chankowsky J, Mullah M, Marcoux J. Placement accuracy of external ventricular drain when comparing freehand insertion to neuronavigation guidance in severe traumatic brain injury. *Acta Neurochir (Wien).* 2017;159(8):1399-1411. doi:10.1007/s00701-017-3201-5.

59. Mahan M, Spetzler RF, Nakaji P. Electromagnetic stereotactic navigation for external ventricular drain placement in the intensive care unit. *J Clin Neurosci.* 2013;20(12):1718-1722. doi:10.1016/j.jocn.2013.03.005.

60. Manfield JH, Yu KKH. Real-time ultrasound-guided external ventricular drain placement. Technical note. *Neurosurg Focus.* 2017;43(5):E5. doi:10.3171/2017.7. FOCUS17148.

61. Wilson TJ, Stetler WR Jr, Al-Holou WN, Sullivan SE. Comparison of the accuracy of ventricular catheter placement using freehand placement, ultrasonic guidance, and stereotactic neuronavigation. *J Neurosurg.* 2013;119(1):66-70. doi:10.3171/2012.11. JNS111384.

62. Eisenring CV, Burn F, Baumann M, et al. sEVD-smartphone-navigated placement of external ventricular drains. *Acta Neurochir (Wien).* 2020;162(3):513-521. doi:10.1007/s00701-019-04131-9.

63. Li Y, Chen X, Wang N, et al. A wearable mixed-reality holographic computer for guiding external ventricular drain insertion at the bedside. *J Neurosurg.* 2018:1-8. doi:10.3171/2018.4.JNS18124.
64. Fiorella D, Peeling L, Denice CM, Sarmiento M, Woo HH. Integrated flat detector CT and live fluoroscopic-guided external ventricular drain placement within the neuroangiography suite. *J Neurointerv Surg.* 2014;6(6):457-460. doi:10.1136/neurintsurg-2013-010856.
65. Roach J, Gaastra B, Bulters D, Shtaya A. Safety, accuracy, and cost effectiveness of bedside bolt external ventricular drains (EVDs) in comparison with tunneled EVDs inserted in theaters. *World Neurosurg.* 2019;125:e473-e478. doi:10.1016/j.wneu.2019.01.106.

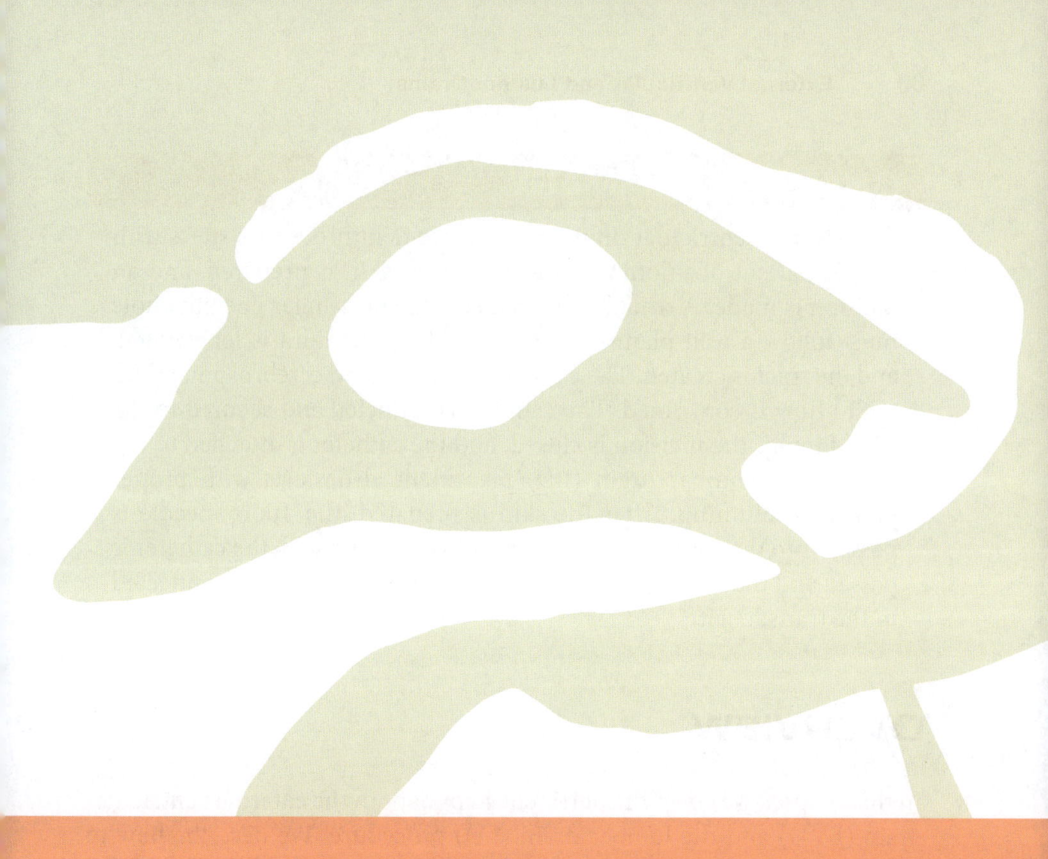

CHAPTER 4

Procedure

CHAPTER SUMMARY

An external ventricular drain (EVD) placement procedure starts with proper patient positioning. Hair is clipped, skin is prepared, and an incision is made. A drill is used to create the burr hole. The burr hole must follow a well-planned trajectory. Next, the dura is fenestrated, and the tract is created. The catheter is passed, and cerebrospinal fluid (CSF) flow is confirmed. The catheter is tunneled and secured to the skin. Finally, the incision is closed, and the catheter is attached to the transducer. Lumbar drain (LD) placement also starts with proper patient positioning. After the skin is prepared, the Tuohy needle is passed into the thecal sac. Once CSF flow is confirmed, the catheter is passed and the needle is removed. The drain is secured and connected to the transducer.

OVERVIEW

In this chapter, we cover the pertinent steps of both the external ventricular drain (EVD) and the lumbar drain (LD) procedure. We describe how to troubleshoot problems that can occur at each point of the procedure, and we review the management of complications. Our intent is to give not only the surgeons but also all other members of the medical team an understanding of what occurs during EVD and LD placement so that each drain can be managed successfully after placement.

PATIENT POSITIONING FOR AN EVD

The patient is positioned for the EVD procedure only after any necessary stabilization. Then, after laboratory workup, medication reversal, and equipment preparation are complete, the patient is positioned for the procedure.

Kocher Point

The Kocher point is the most commonly used approach, as introduced in Chap. 2 ("Anatomy"). If the EVD is being placed at the bedside and in an urgent or emergent manner, the Kocher point should always be used. Its use requires the patient to be positioned supine, with the head in a neutral position. Care should be taken to avoid extending the head, and even slight flexion may be helpful. Extension of the head will bring the exit point of the tunneling trocar closer to the head of the bed, thus increasing the difficulty in exiting the skin. The head of the bed can initially remain elevated to 30° or more (Fig. 4.1). Once the head of the bed has been elevated, the head of the patient should be secured. Some surgeons secure the patient's head to the bed using tape across the patient's forehead. However, we have moved away from this practice because we have found that having a second person hold the head steady is more stable than tape. Tape also can induce some extension, especially if the patient sinks lower in the bed, which, as noted previously, can be problematic.

Other Entry Points

Any entry point described in Chap. 2, other than the Kocher point, is likely to be used only in the operating room, where the EVD may or may not

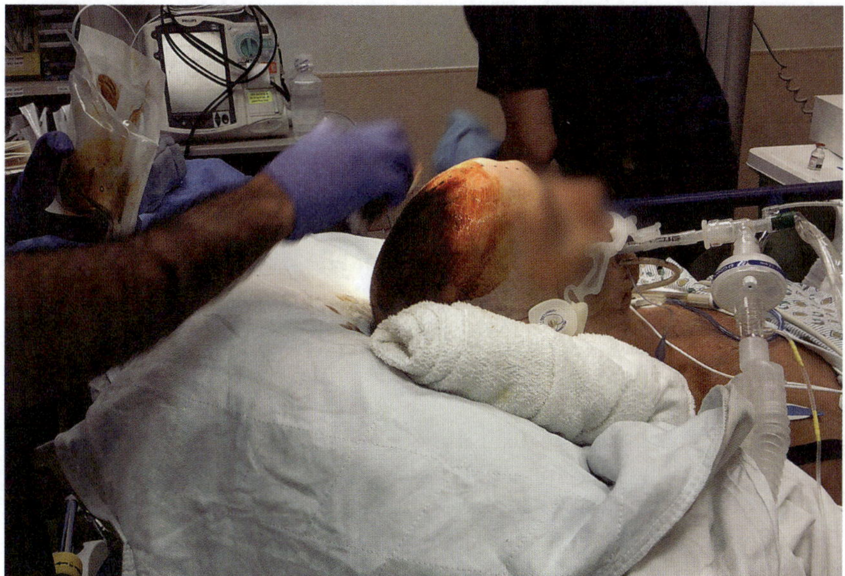

FIGURE 4.1. Skin preparation. After hair clipping, scalp cleansing, and marking of the appropriate landmarks, the sterilizing solution is applied to the site. In this case, an iodine-based solution was used. The application of the sterilizing solution is started at the center of the incision, and an outward circular motion is used to coat the entire area. This process is repeated multiple times, and the solution is allowed to air-dry according to the manufacturer's recommendations. During this part of the procedure, the head of the bed can remain elevated to 30°, which is especially important in patients with increased intracranial pressure. A rolled towel rather than tape is used to maintain the head in a neutral position. Note the electrocardiogram sticker marking the location of the tragus.

be part of a larger cranial procedure. Use of another entry point requires thoughtful planning, as well as the incorporation of a Mayfield clamp. Whether the patient will receive the EVD before or after the cranial procedure or must be discussed. The Barrow point may be best accessed with the patient supine, with a slight bump placed underneath the ipsilateral shoulder, and the head turned fully to the contralateral side. The Keen point is accessed with the patient in the same position. If an EVD is placed intraoperatively, patient positioning is dictated by the craniotomy. The midline posterior approaches, which allow access to the Frazier and Dandy points, are completed with the patient prone and in a head clamp, with the head slightly flexed and the chin tucked. These approaches can also be completed with the patient in the lateral or three-quarters lateral position, with flexion of the head and the nose of the patient turned down toward the floor to the contralateral side. In all cases, especially if a longer craniotomy procedure is being planned, adequate padding should be ensured.

EVD PROCEDURE: STEPS, NUANCES, AND COMPLICATION MANAGEMENT

Skin Preparation

The EVD procedure covered in the following sections is for a Kocher entry point, which begins with cutting the patient's hair. Electric clippers should be used rather than a razor, and care should be taken to avoid nicking the skin. The surgeon should confirm that the shaving is being done on the correct side. None of the authors have adopted a policy of minimal cutting of the hair for EVDs. A more exposed scalp allows better adhesion of the drape of the craniotomy kit, better adhesion of the dressing at the end of the procedure, easier identification of a cerebrospinal fluid (CSF) leak from the incision, and easier removal of sutures or staples after the incision has healed. We shave enough hair to expose the midline laterally to the superior temporal line and posteriorly enough to allow for the exit of the tunneling trocar.

Next, an initial round of scalp cleaning is performed (Fig. 4.1). Cleansing is focused on the exposed scalp, as well as the surrounding hair. It can be done with soap and water, surgical scrub sponges, or any combination of sterilizing solutions. Once the scalp is dry, a sterile marker is used to delineate the appropriate landmarks and entry point. Points marked include the midline, a point 10 to 11 cm from the nasion, and a point 2 to 3 cm from the midline. Some surgeons may choose to mark the hairline, the location of the coronal suture as palpated through the skin, and the midpupillary line. We prefer to press the tip of the marker into the skin at the entry point, which prevents loss of the mark during the sterile scrub. At this point, the surgeon should confirm yet again that the markings are on the correct side. We place an electrocardiogram sticker on both the ipsilateral tragus and the nasion of the patient so that the metal nub can be palpated beneath the sterile drapes.

The CSF collection chamber is prepared and mounted on a pole, with the proximal tubing kept sterile (Fig. 4.2A). The pressure transduction chamber is opened, as are the sterile red caps. Sterile gloves are donned, and the pressure transducer is attached to the collection chamber. A sterile normal saline syringe is opened, and the pressure transducer is flushed simultaneously, as a red cap is placed at the end (Fig. 4.2B). Next, the three-way stopcock on the collection chamber is manipulated to flush the proximal line until saline emanates from the end. The distal line is then flushed into the collection chamber. The pressure transducer cable is attached, and the entire system is set aside (Fig. 4.2C).

The surgeon ensures for the last time that all the necessary equipment and staff are present. Next, the access kit is opened and the towels, sutures, and EVD catheter are dropped in a sterile fashion onto the surgical field. The surgeon dons a surgical cap, a face mask, an eye shield, a sterile gown, and two pairs of sterile gloves. A sterilizing solution is then applied to the scalp of the patient. A 2015 Cochrane Review[1] and other reports have found that chlorhexidine-based solutions are better than other methods at reducing the rate of surgical site infections.[1,2] The scrub is started over the incision, then moved outward in concentric circles to the periphery where the hair is untrimmed. We perform the sterilization process twice, each time using a new sterile solution applicator and allowing the solution to completely dry between applications. Once the site is dry, a sterile marker and ruler are used to re-mark all the previously drawn lines without contaminating the sterile gloves. The incision is marked to be no less than 3 cm long. We have not adapted the stab incision technique for tunneled EVDs because it increases the difficulty and the risk of damaging or pulling the catheter when using the tunneling trocar. It also increases the risk of damaging the catheter when grabbing the galea on closure. Next, the patient is draped. The sterile towels are placed in a specific order. The midline towel is placed first, exposing the midline mark and the edge of the unclipped hair. Next, the inferior towel is placed across the pillow or the head of the bed, making sure to leave enough room for the exit point of the trocar (Fig. 4.3A). Then the lateral towel is placed at the edge of the shaved hair, covering the patient's ear. Depending on how many towels are in the pack,

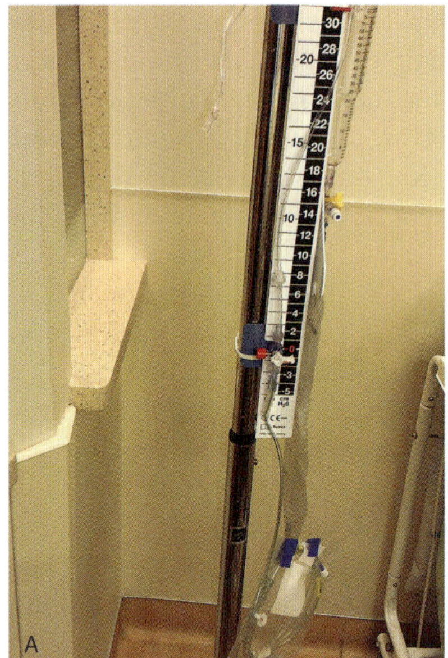
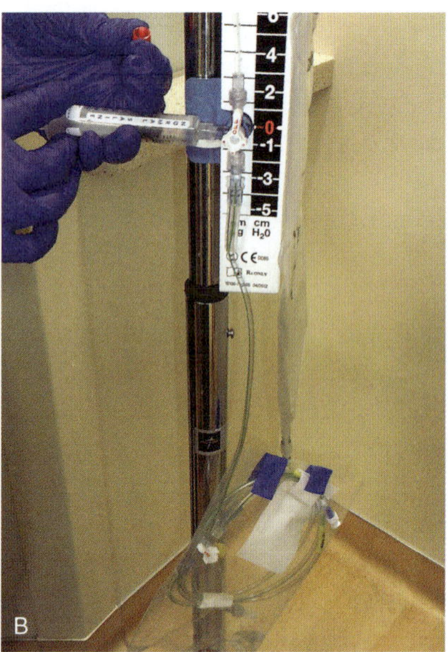
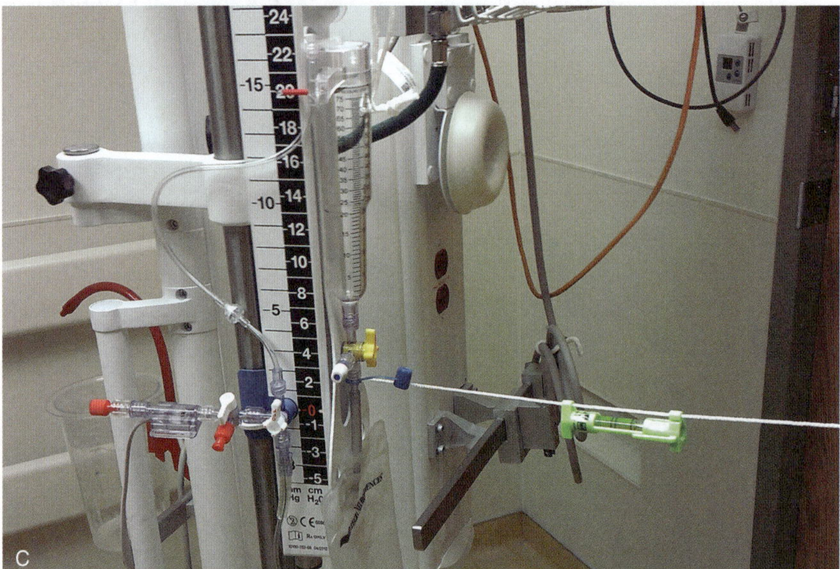

FIGURE 4.2. Collection chamber setup. **A.** The collection chamber is attached to the pole. **B.** The system is flushed both proximally and distally. **C.** The pressure transducer and leveling indicator are attached.

one is placed superior and frontally to cover the patient's forehead and eyes. A final towel is placed off to the left or right of the head of the patient, depending on where the rest of the equipment is located, to cover the head

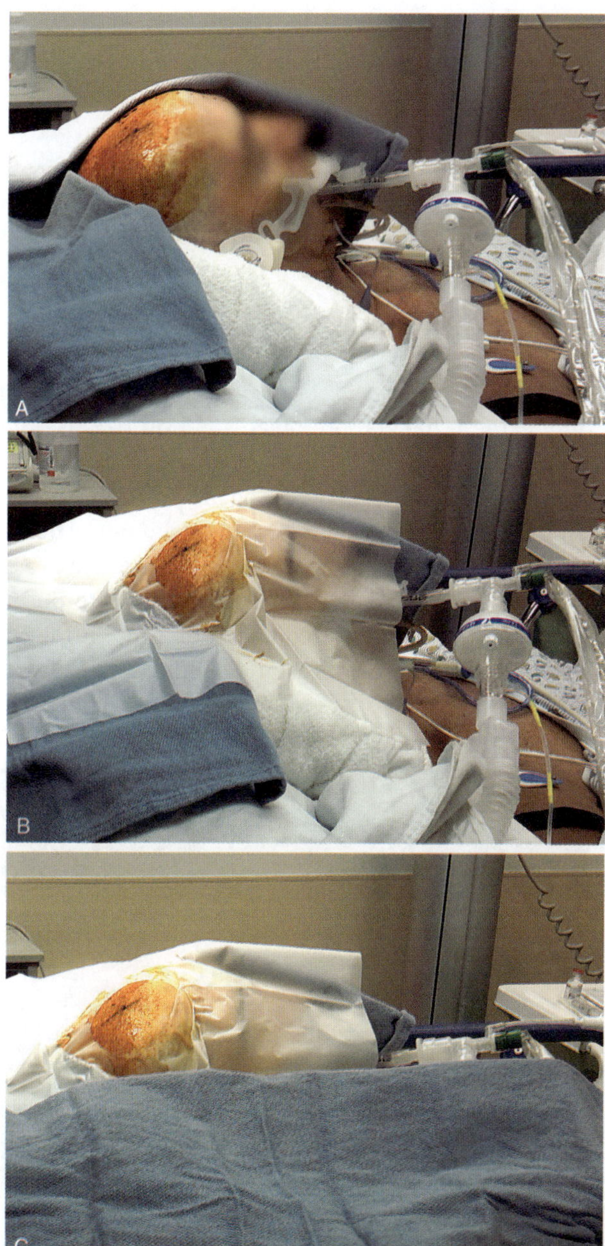

FIGURE 4.3. Draping for the external ventricular drain procedure. **A.** Draping is initiated, with the first towel alongside the midline marker. The second towel is the inferior one placed across the pillow to afford some protection by establishing the sterile field. **B.** Next the clear plastic drape can be placed. **C.** We recommend expanding the sterile field as much as possible to give the surgeon maximal working room. This can be done with additional sterile towels or a half drape placed inferiorly.

of the bed and increase the sterile field. Finally, the plastic drape with the precut hole that comes standard in the kit is placed over the incision site (Fig. 4.3B). A sterile half drape covers the head of the bed to expand the sterile field and give the surgeon maximal working room (Fig. 4.3C).

Just before the incision is made, a surgical time-out is taken by everyone in the room. This break in the action allows us to confirm that we have the correct patient, procedure, site, side, and indications. We also review documented allergies and other relevant patient history.

Skin Incision

The skin is infiltrated with sterile lidocaine solution. We prefer to use epinephrine–lidocaine 1:200,000 premixed solution because the epinephrine gives the added vasoconstrictive effect to reduce skin edge bleeding, and it prolongs the effect of the analgesic agent.[3] We infiltrate both superficially in the loose connective tissue layer and deep in the periosteal layer to form a large welt, which has the added benefit of pressure to tamponade bleeding from scalp arteries (Fig. 4.4). We also infiltrate the tract of the tunneling trocar, which is then allowed to set for 2 or 3 minutes for maximal effect. During this time, the assistant administers the perioperative antibiotics and any additional doses of sedative and analgesic medication

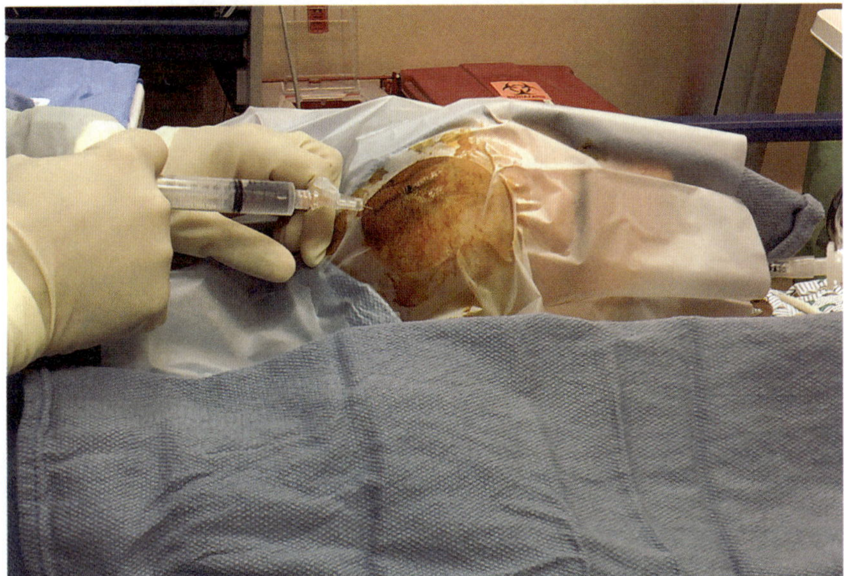

FIGURE 4.4. Local anesthetic. After a surgical time-out to double-check the patient and confirm the procedure, the skin incision site and the trocar track are infiltrated with a local anesthetic.

(eg, fentanyl, midazolam, propofol) to prepare the patient. The rest of the access kit is also prepared during this time.

You should check the drill, retractor, forceps, scissors, hemostats, and needle driver to ensure that they are functional, and the drill bit, needles, and knives to ensure that they are sharp. Place the safety stop on the drill bit. Lay out the instruments in their order of use, and fill the tray bottom with sterile saline (Fig. 4.5). Remove the stylet of the EVD catheter, and place the clear plastic adapter in the catheter set loosely on the end of the catheter. Flush the catheter once with sterile saline before placing the stylet back through the catheter with the plastic cap still on, then set aside the catheter.

To start the incision, position the tip of the blade at the top of the incision, and take the blade down to the bone. Cut the rest of the incision at this depth with the belly of the blade, taking care not to use a sawing action or skiving. Use the back of the blade to strip the periosteum on each side of the incision. At this point, you may encounter some bleeding from the skin. Use a small retractor to control the bleeding, which is sufficient in most cases. Place the retractor with the handle facing upward toward the patient's forehead, so that it spreads the incision at least to the depth of the galea (Fig. 4.6).

You will inevitably encounter bleeding from a scalp artery, a terminal branch of the temporal artery, or a frontal branch of the superficial temporal artery that is not controllable with either the lidocaine welt or the

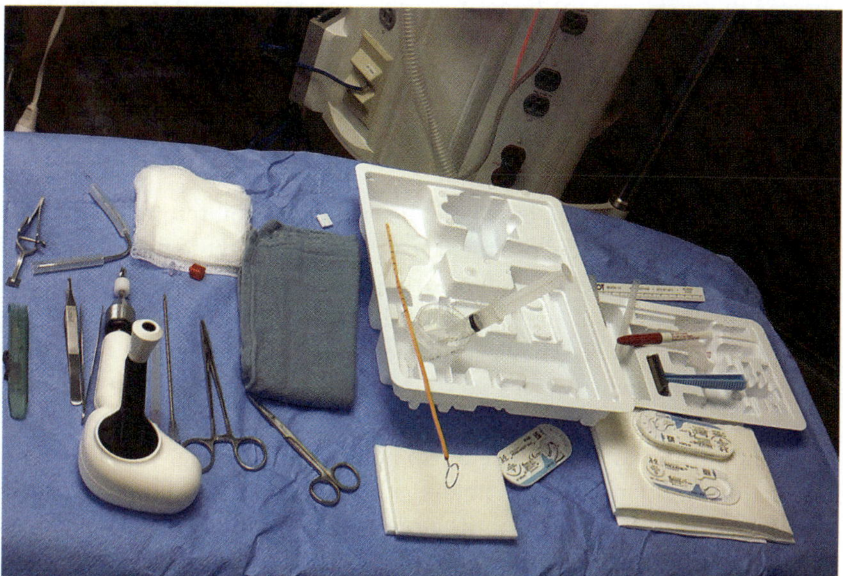

FIGURE 4.5. Kit preparation. The external ventricular drain kit equipment is inventoried, prepared, and laid out in its order of use while the local anesthetic activates.

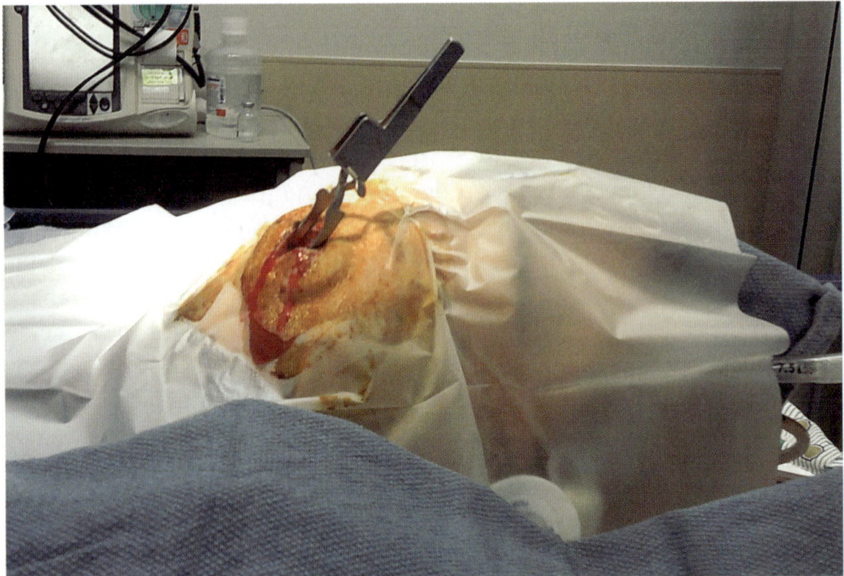

FIGURE 4.6. Retractor. After the skin is excised and the periosteum is peeled off the skull, a small retractor is inserted with its blades underneath the galea. We prefer to place the retractor so that the handle points away from the surgeon and does not interfere with the rest of the procedure.

insertion of the retractor. This bleeding will quickly fill the incision and obscure the surface of the bone. You can place a gauze pad in the incision and hold it there for a minute, or you can use a hemostat to pinch the artery closed then set the tool aside.

Burr Hole

It is now time to make the burr hole. Insert the drill bit into the drill until it meets the bottom, and close the three prongs around the bit as tightly as possible by holding the head of the drill in place with one palm and rotating the circular arm of the drill with the other hand. Double-check the security of the drill bit. The head of the bed can be lowered at this point to be nearly flat, which gives you a better working angle. The assistant then reaches underneath the sterile towels to clasp the head of the patient alongside each ear, cradling the jaw to hold it in place (Fig. 4.7). Place the drill bit on the bone surface, holding the handle in the dominant hand (Fig. 4.8). The metallic nubs of the electrocardiogram stickers underneath the drapes indicate the nasion and ipsilateral tragus.

The location where lines directed inward from these two points intersect is roughly the location of the ipsilateral foramen of Monro, and is the

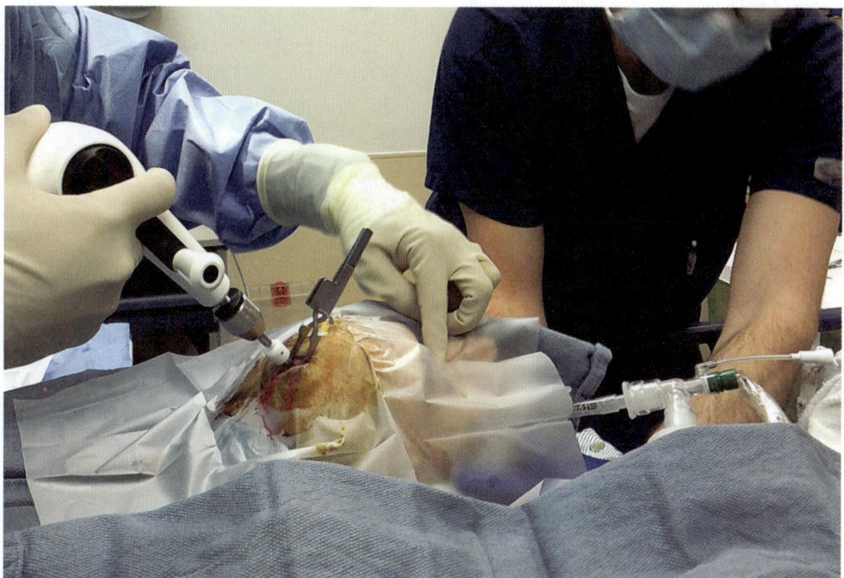

FIGURE 4.7. Head stabilization. The surgeon palpates the necessary landmarks to ensure that the trajectory is correct before starting to drill. An assistant reaches underneath the drape to hold the patient steady, as needed.

target for the trajectory you will follow. Some authors argue for an orthogonal approach to the bone and the elimination of trajectories; the orthogonal approach has been shown to be equivalent in a systematic review, and the ipsilateral medial canthus was found to be inferior in simulation trials.[4] Because the drill bit is only slightly larger than the catheter, the trajectory of the burr hole can affect the final trajectory. Ultimately, the trajectory is partially an internal reference that you will build over time and partially a combination of factors such as the midline shift. We start with the drill orthogonal at first and rotate it quickly but in a controlled manner just above the point of contact. Starting at a low speed with direct contact almost guarantees that the drill bit will "jump" off the bone and down the side, causing loss of both the entry point and the trajectory. The failure to recognize this slip is one of the most common errors that leads to an unsuccessful drain placement. An alternative technique is to start with a slow rotation of the drill and create a notch by returning to the same place each time the bit skips off.

Once enough of a notch has been created in the outer cortical layer, the drill bit will not slip and only the trajectory must be kept in mind. The drill can be kept orthogonal or adjusted to the desired trajectory. As the drilling continues, you should keep a high rate of rotation and apply moderate downward pressure. The outer cortex of the bone will offer considerable

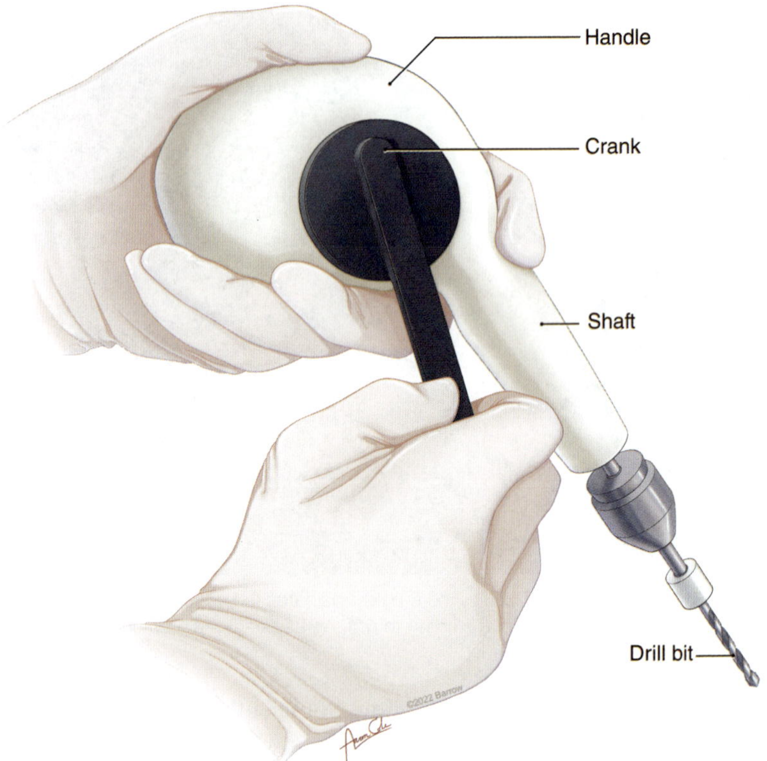

FIGURE 4.8. Proper handling of the hand drill. Artist's illustration demonstrates the proper technique for holding the hand-operated drill. The left-hand fingers and palm grip the base of the drill, while the right-hand fingers grip the turn-crank.

resistance, which will lessen once the diploic space is entered. When the inner cortex is reached, resistance will again be encountered. You should then lighten the downward pressure to avoid plunging the drill bit into the brain when the inner cortex is broken. There is a fine balance between the forward rotation of the drill and your slight backward pull on the drill. The drill bit may almost feel as if it is stuck, but it can be continued forward. Once the inner cortex is broken, you will experience a suction-like feeling and noise that will pull the drill forward. You must then keep the drill bit rotating forward but pull it out with backward pressure (Fig. 4.9).

Once the drill bit is removed from the burr hole, we prefer to irrigate the hole with sterile saline to clear the surgical field. There is usually some bleeding (Fig. 4.10). At times the bleeding can be quite brisk, but it is almost never serious and nothing more than a bony venous channel. Any bleeding at this stage is always cleared with irrigation only. Avoid placing

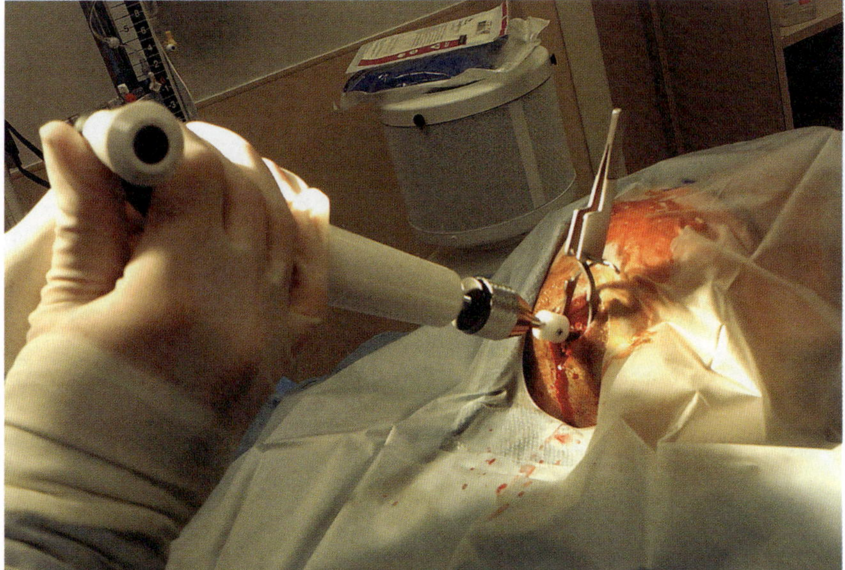

FIGURE 4.9. Drilling. As the drilling process nears the inner cortical bone, the hand position changes. The left hand pulls the handle back, while the right-hand fingers continue to spin the drill clockwise and forward in a controlled fashion until the drill is felt to "pull in" toward the brain.

a piece of gauze in the hole to tamponade the bleeding because doing so can inadvertently lead to the blood collecting epidurally. In a few cases, we have had to use more than a liter of normal saline irrigation to slow the bleeding. Forceps should also not be used to grab bone chips from the burr hole because doing so may lodge some pieces underneath the cortex.

The drill bit has also been known to come loose from its prongs during the drilling. This happens because even slight reverse rotation will loosen the drill bit when it is snugly caught in the bone. The drill bit is simply placed back in the prongs of the drill, which is tightened it as it was when first placed. Thereafter, you must use only forward rotation. Alternatively, you can rotate the entire drill as a unit by holding the rotating arm in place and rotating the handle in the forward direction. Doing so may seem awkward at first, but it may be helpful in this setting. We have never had a drill bit break rather than come loose; however, in a case of a broken drill bit, depending on how much bit remains protruding from the bone, you can try gripping the protruding bit with the prongs of the drill head to remove it. Otherwise, a craniotomy may be required. Depending on how critical the patient is, a second burr hole may be made to pass the drain from the same incision before proceeding to a craniotomy to remove the drill bit.

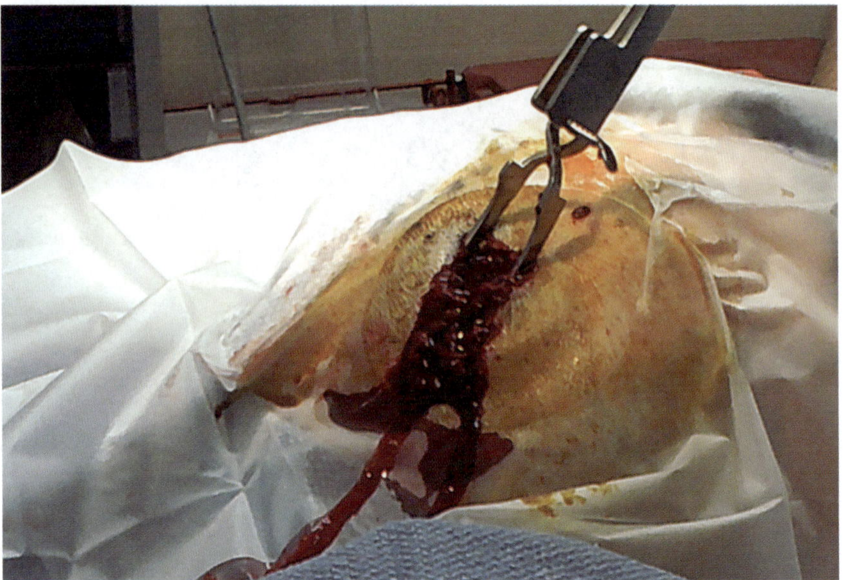

FIGURE 4.10. Bleeding. Drilling usually results in some degree of bleeding. Hemorrhage occurs most often from the bone edges or the venous lacunae within the bone. It can be managed with continued irrigation until the bleeding slows. Every effort should be made not to plug the hole with a sponge because doing so may drive the bleeding intracranially as an epidural or a subdural hemorrhage.

Passing the Catheter

After the burr hole has been placed, we tunnel the trocar. Tunneling requires bending the trocar to nearly a 90° angle at its midpoint. Keep the protective covering on the trocar and grab only the back end of it to fulcrum the anterior half on the table. Once the trocar is bent, remove the front protective cap. Use extreme care with the trocar because it is extremely sharp. Use the forceps to lift the skin at the incision site and the galea, then pass the front of the trocar underneath the galea (Fig. 4.11A). Passing the trocar above the galea may cause the skin to tear, eventually requiring it to be sutured. We prefer to aim the trocar posteriorly and medially. The exit site may require modification if a craniotomy incision will be made after EVD placement. Grab the back of the trocar with a needle driver, then push and guide it to its exit point. We attempt to make the exit site at least 5 cm away from the incision. This process can be painful, so the patient should be adequately medicated. A hemostat is used to provide counter resistance on the skin at the exit site. When the tip of the trocar protrudes from the skin, grab it with the needle driver (Fig. 4.11B). The 90° bend in the trocar will help prevent it from passing through the towels into the bed. Extreme care should be taken

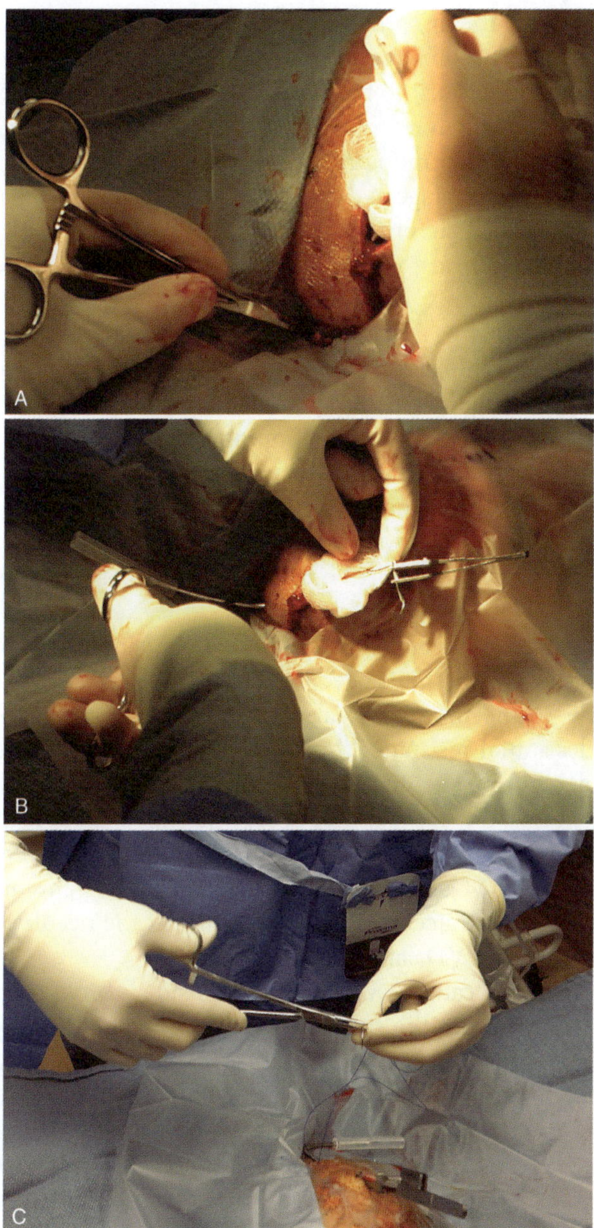

FIGURE 4.11. Passing the trocar. **A.** The trocar is passed after it has been bent. The skin and galea are lifted, and the sharp end is pushed to an exit point 5 cm from the bony entrance. Counterpressure on the skin is provided with a long instrument to help safely exit the skin. **B.** After the sharp end of the trocar has protruded, a clamp is used to pull it through, while the other hand pushes gently on the ribbed end. The bend in the trocar facilitates its exit away from the drape. The sharp end should be capped as soon as enough of the tip is exposed. **C.** The exit site suture can be passed at this point because hitting the metal trocar is inconsequential.

when maneuvering the tip, which should be covered with the protective cap as soon as possible. In some cases, the patient will move during this process, causing the tip of the trocar to penetrate not only its protective cap but also both surgical gloves and the surgeon's hand, which has been my (R.R.) experience in one case. A common practice is to now throw the suture securing the exit point. The advantage of doing so is that the bite can be full thickness and close to the exit hole of the trocar without jeopardizing the catheter, which is the main concern when suturing is done later (Fig. 4.11C). Tuck the back end of the trocar underneath the retractor blade. Point the front end away from the surgical field until the trocar is needed again.

With the trocar in place, use a spinal needle to fenestrate the dura in a circular motion along the periphery of the burr hole. Each time the needle pierces the dura, you should feel a popping sensation. Refrain from passing the needle too far down after the popping sensation because doing so increases the risk of injuring the underlying cortical vessels. The needle will also allow you to detect whether the deep rim of the burr hole has been evenly cut. If a lip exists, the drill must be brought in again to even out the inner opening.

After the dura has been fenestrated, use a Cushing needle to break the fenestration (Fig. 4.12A). This needle is wide and blunt. Once it is placed in the burr hole, the needle should take the same trajectory as the EVD. The dura provides initial resistance, but it will also eventually give way with a popping sensation (Fig. 4.12B). If advancing the dural needle requires considerable force, the dura has not been fenestrated enough, and another round of fenestration with the long needle is needed. Once the dural hole has been created, the Cushing needle is advanced 2 to 3 cm into the brain after confirming the trajectory. This advancing of the needle is helpful to create a tract for the EVD catheter to follow.

Finally, the EVD catheter with the stylet inside is brought into the surgical field. Confirm that the stylet has been pushed all the way to the tip of the catheter. Hold the catheter with your dominant hand at approximately the 6-cm mark between your thumb and index finger. After reconfirming the trajectory, pass the catheter (Fig. 4.13A). There may be a "ribbing" sensation initially, which is caused by the catheter holes rubbing against the bone edge and may feel similar to running your hand against ribs in the chest wall. A little initial resistance is normal. Excessive resistance may indicate that the dura has not been fully fenestrated and more work is needed. When the catheter enters the ventricle, you will feel a gentle popping sensation or a loss of resistance (Fig. 4.13B). Depending on the pressure inside the ventricle, CSF may emanate from the top of the catheter. If this occurs, usually at around 5 cm, remove the stylet while keeping the

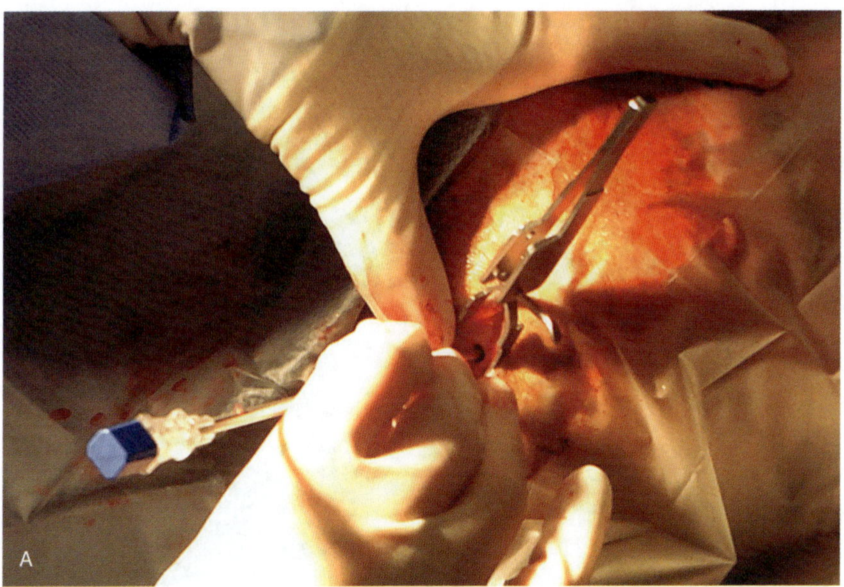

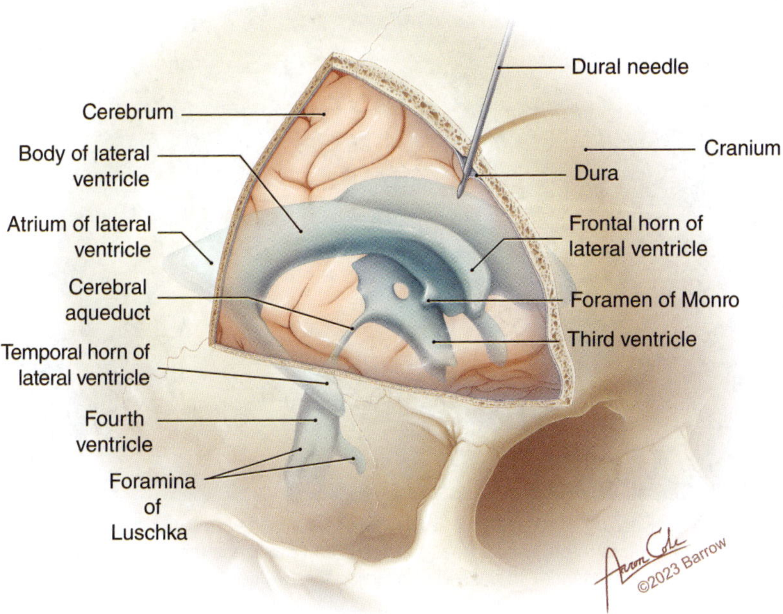

FIGURE 4.12. Needle passing through the dura. **A.** The Cushing dural needle is used to break through the circular dural fenestration made with the spinal needle. **B.** The dural needle will encounter resistance until it enters through the dura. Artist's illustration demonstrates the dural needle entering the dura.

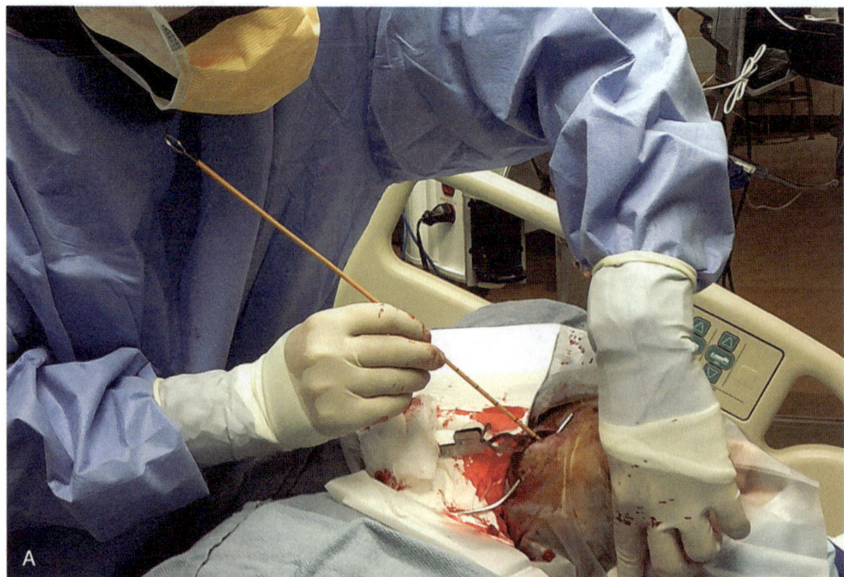

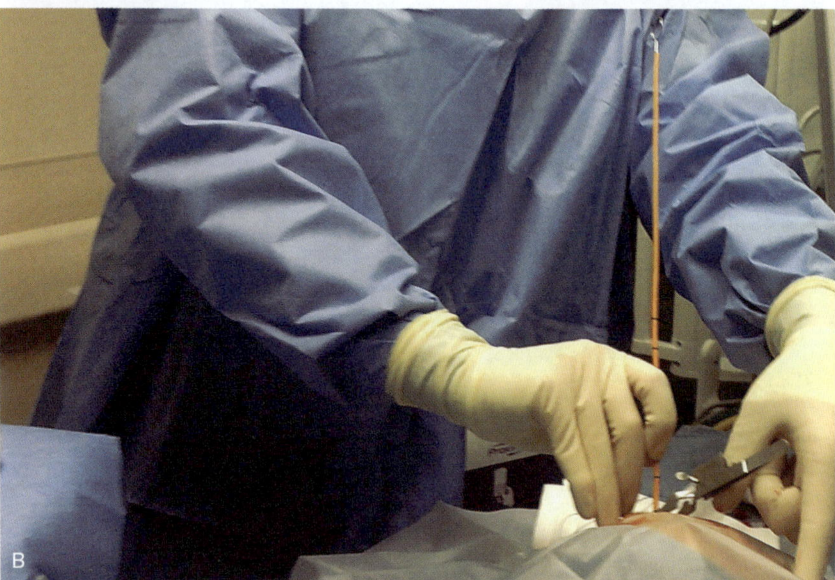

FIGURE 4.13. Passing the catheter. **A.** With the catheter in the burr hole, the landmarks are noted. **B.** The catheter is then passed slowly, taking care to process the sensations in the fingertips as different tissue planes are passed and feeling for the "pop" sensed upon entering the ventricle. **C.** When the surgeon believes that the catheter is in the ventricle, the stylet is removed and cerebrospinal fluid flow is assessed. **D.** Artist's illustration demonstrates the catheter being soft passed to no deeper than 7 cm with its final resting place in the foramen of Monro.

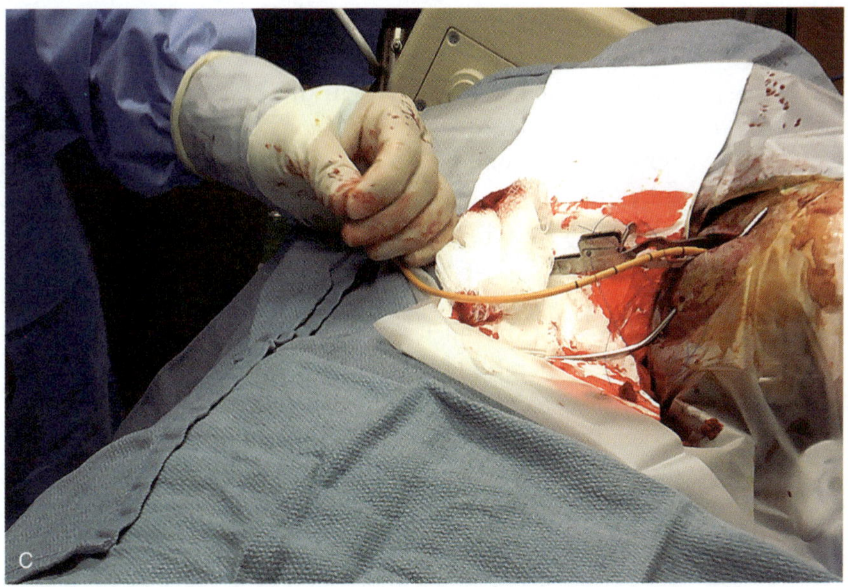

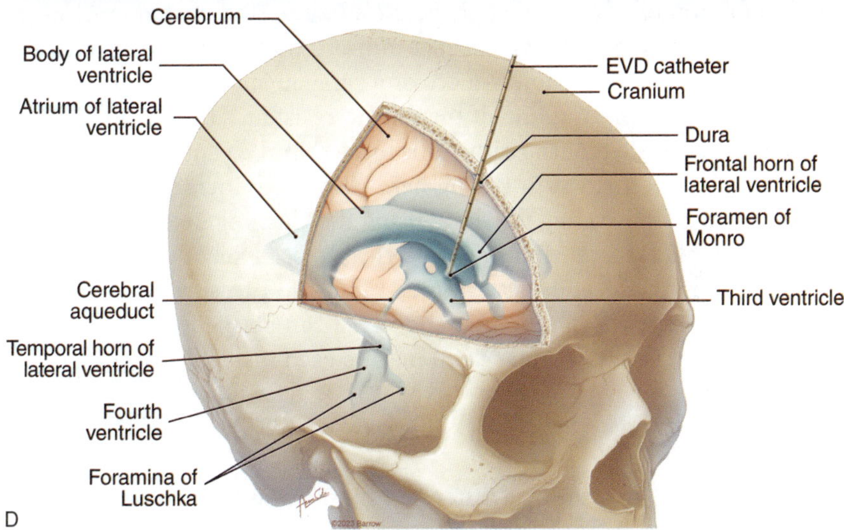

FIGURE 4.13. (Continued)

catheter steady (Fig. 4.13C). Temporarily occlude the catheter between the thumb and index finger and "soft pass" it 1 cm until your thumb meets the bone surface. Check for CSF flow again, and place the red cap on the clear plastic adapter. At each check for CSF flow, a minimal amount of CSF is released. Figure 4.13D illustrates the final depth of the catheter at the skull surface.

A gentle increase in resistance as your thumb reaches the bone surface at the 6-cm mark may be an indication that the trajectory is wrong, and the catheter is in the basal ganglia or caudate. In this case, no CSF will flow. However, there are instances of the catheter being placed in the ventricle without a CSF flow. This lack of flow can happen when pressure in the ventricle is low or the catheter is air-locked. If the catheter reaches 6 cm and no CSF flows, keep the position at the skull fixed and drop the end of the catheter below head height. If this maneuver does not prove successful, your next move is to break the air lock if such exists. Use a syringe from the EVD kit with the plunger removed. Attach the syringe to the plastic adapter at the end of the catheter. Then fill the syringe with sterile saline and, while holding the catheter in a fixed position at the skull, raise the syringe end as far above the head as possible without pulling out the catheter. If the catheter is inside the ventricle, the level of saline will drop. Lower the hand holding the syringe, which causes the syringe to fill back up in a process known as tidaling. Removing the syringe should result in CSF flow. If this technique is still not successful, attach the plunger to the syringe filled with a small amount of saline and apply gentle suction. If there is no resistance and fluid is easily withdrawn, it may indicate that the catheter is in the ventricle. Only if this suction is successful can you apply gentle pressure to inject less than 1 mL of saline. If there is no resistance to the saline injection, it may indicate that the catheter is located in the ventricle.

A final caution is worth noting here. Any brisk increase in bleeding, whether while fenestrating the dura, using the Cushing needle, or passing the catheter, may indicate injury to a cortical vessel, likely a vein. As before, the key to control bleeding is continued irrigation to slow it. If bleeding persists, an attempt to tamponade the vessel can be made by passing the catheter. Alternatively, a cautery pen may be used inside the burr hole.

Closure

With the catheter in place, your attention should now be focused on finishing the procedure. It is critical to protect the catheter at all times. First, pull the clear plastic adapter with the red cap off the end of the catheter, and pinch the catheter to temporarily occlude it. Expose the back of the trocar hidden underneath the retractor blade, and load the end of the catheter onto it. We suggest putting the end of the catheter at least past the third ribbing on the end of the trocar because the catheter can become disconnected when pulling through. Use a needle driver to grab the front of the trocar behind the protective cap and pull the catheter through the subgaleal tunnel. With your other hand, grab the catheter with a nontoothed forceps right at the burr hole to prevent it from moving. There will be resistance to pulling the catheter through, but sustained effort will prove successful. Near the end of the pull through, a loop is created by the catheter at the burr hole (Fig. 4.14A). Slightly ease the grip of the hand holding the catheter at the burr hole to allow the catheter to rotate in place and unwind the loop (Fig. 4.14B). Pay careful attention to ensure that the catheter does not advance while rotating. If it does, pulling slightly with the trocar will bring the catheter to the appropriate depth (Fig. 4.14C). Pinch the catheter with one hand to occlude it near the trocar end, and use scissors to cut the catheter at the end of the trocar (Fig. 4.14D). Confirm the flow of CSF (Fig. 4.14E). Fully reattach the clear plastic adapter with the red cap to the end of the catheter (Fig. 4.14F).

With the catheter passed, the next step is to secure it at the skin exit site. Securing the catheter is accomplished with a purse-string technique using 2-0 nylon. If this suture was already passed when the trocar was placed, it will only require tightening around the catheter. If it was not, then the most important part of the suturing now is to prevent inadvertent puncture of the catheter. We enter at the bottom right of the exit site and pass the needle parallel to the tract of the catheter, coming out a half-centimeter above. We then cross over the tract of the catheter and enter at the top left of the exit site, traveling parallel to the tract for 5 mm before exiting at the bottom left. Pull the suture through so there is equal length on both sides, and cut off the needle. Make a tight square knot that gathers the skin around the exit site. If this suture is too snug, it may occlude flow. Cross the ends of the suture over the catheter, then tie a snug square knot on the catheter itself. Repeat this process up the length of the catheter for 5 to 7 knots (Fig. 4.15). The suture and knots should be snug around the catheter but not occlusive. As you make each knot, remove the red cap from the end of the catheter to check CSF flow.

Next, the incision is irrigated with sterile saline. Load another 2-0 nylon suture and start the incision closure. We use a running technique, starting at the very beginning of the incision. Removing the retractor will allow you to observe each bite (Fig. 4.16). Each bite should be started with the needle point perpendicular to the skin, and it should be deep enough to grab galea. Failure to grab and close galea may lead to a CSF leak from the incision. The running stitch is not pulled tight until the end, which allows the incision to remain slack enough to visualize the catheter and galea with each bite.

Some additional points of caution are needed here. First, the catheter can be pulled out when the trocar is being pulled through the skin. If the catheter comes completely out, then it will have to be passed again. If it

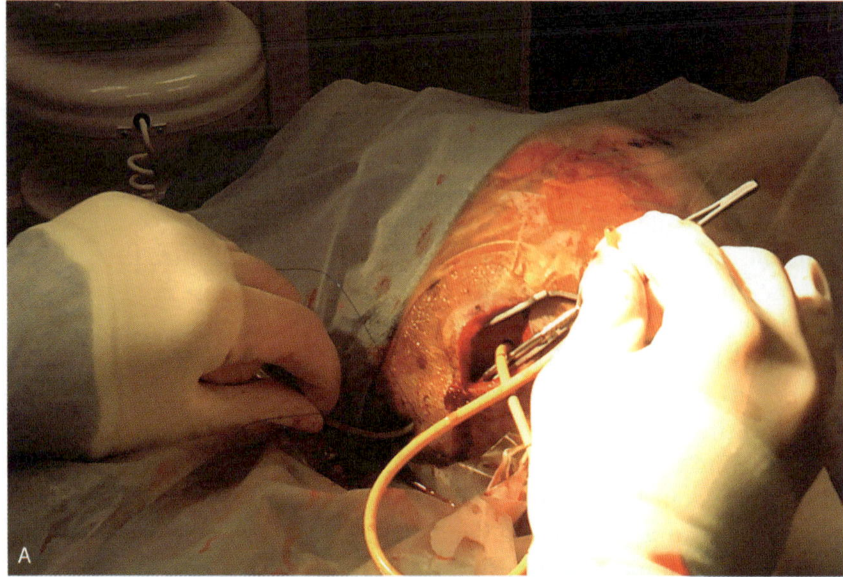

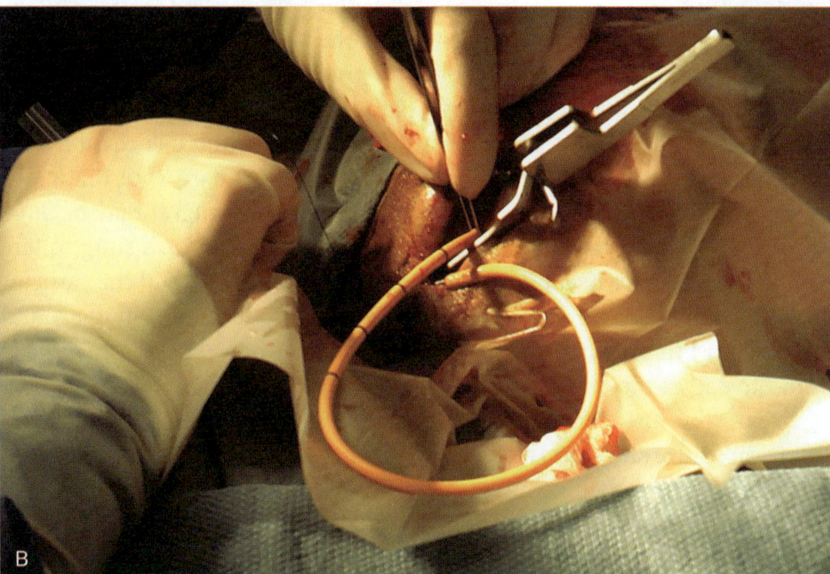

FIGURE 4.14. Tunneling the catheter. **A.** The catheter is confirmed to have cerebrospinal fluid (CSF) flow and is attached to the ribbed end of the trocar. **B.** A nontoothed forceps is used to hold the catheter at the bone exit site in one hand while the other hand begins to pull the trocar from the skin exit site. **C.** The catheter may loop, and care must be taken so that it does not get caught on anything or rotate and enter deeper upon rotation. **D.** The catheter is cut just past the ribbed end of the trocar. **E.** CSF flow is again confirmed. **F.** The clear plastic connector with a red cap is attached to the catheter.

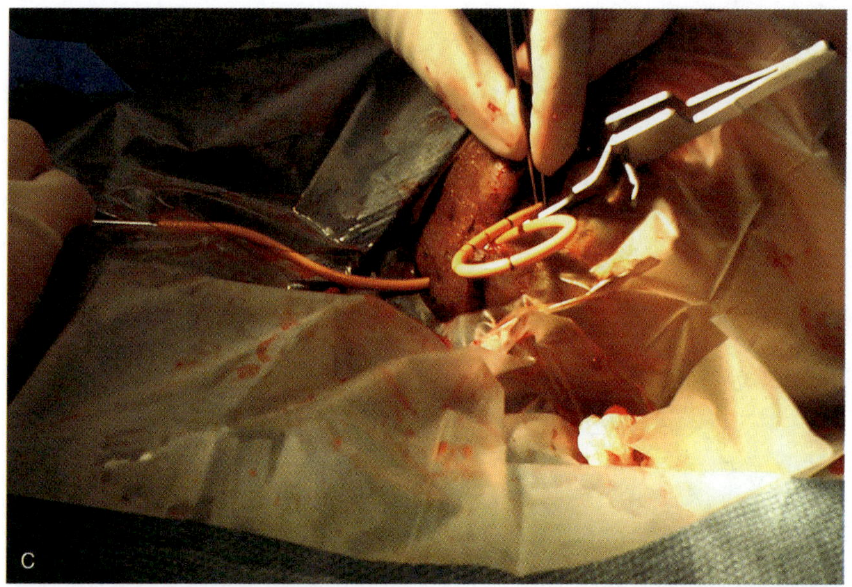

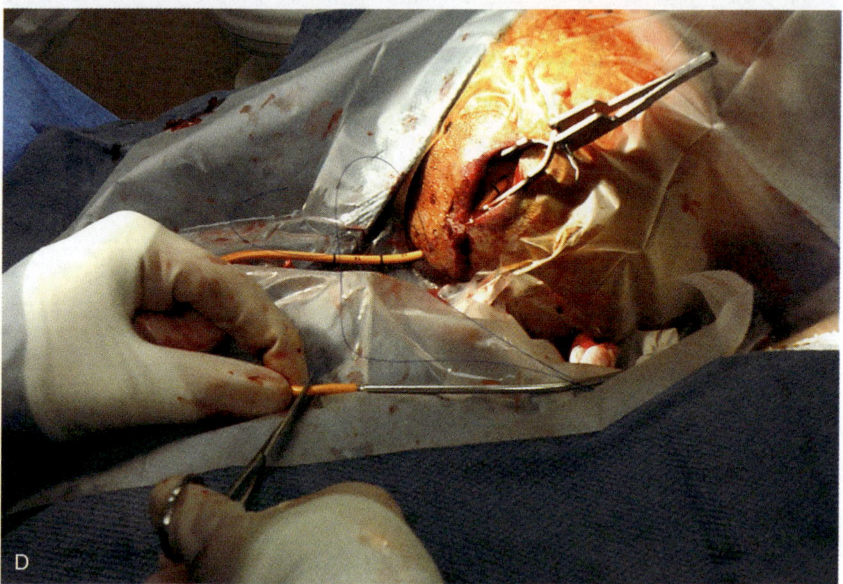

FIGURE 4.14. (Continued)

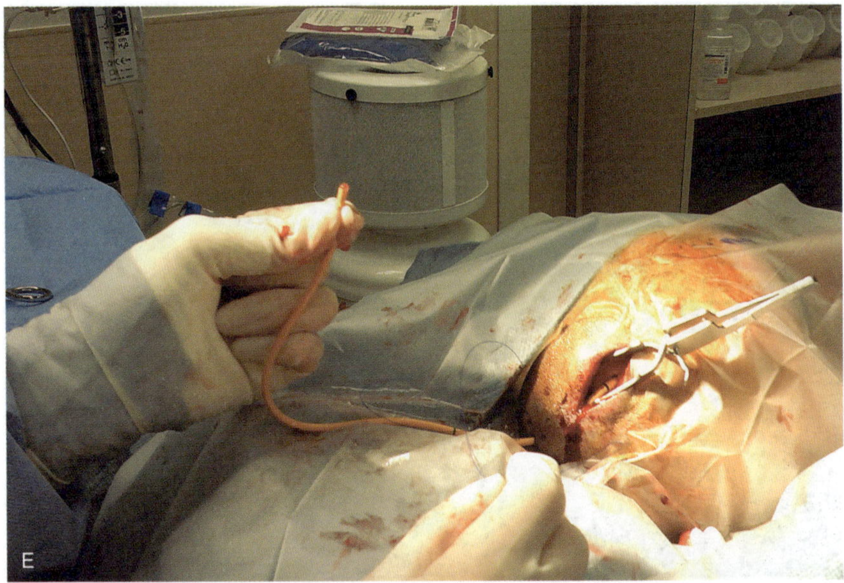

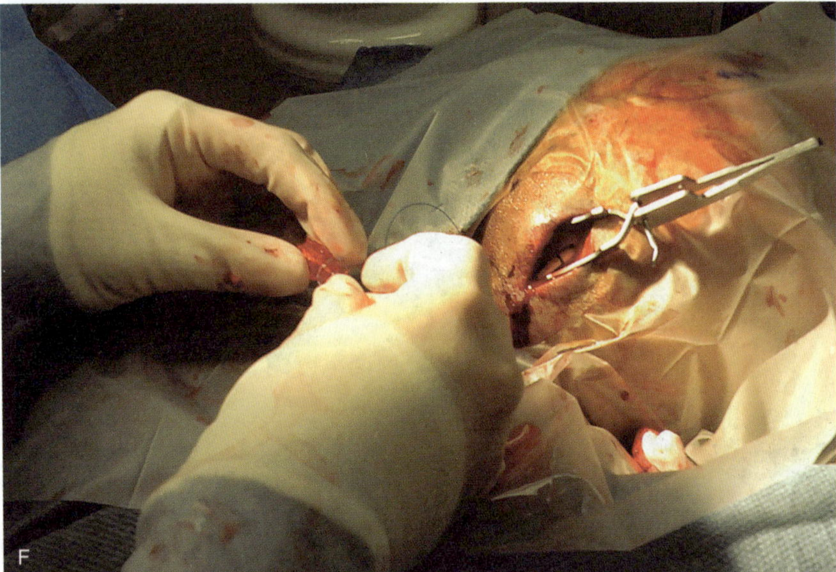

FIGURE 4.14. (Continued)

moves only a small distance, it can be soft passed deeper to its original depth by pulling in slack from the skin. The most worrisome concern is possible damage to the catheter by the needle. Even the smallest puncture spells the end of the catheter because it will induce a CSF leak. A damaged catheter must be removed and replaced with a new one. Although we

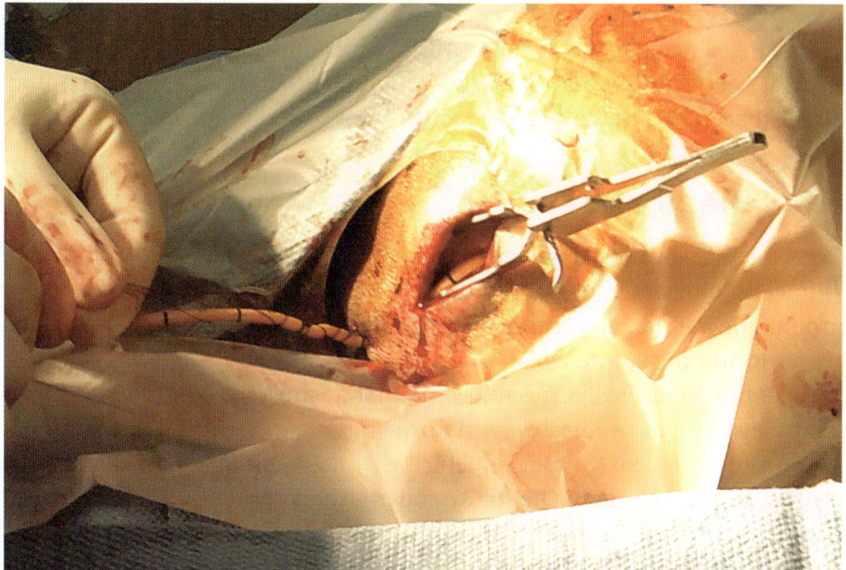

FIGURE 4.15. Securing the catheter. The suture at the skin exit site is tied along the catheter. The knots should be tight enough to grip the catheter but not so tight as to occlude the catheter. Note the waistband appearance of a properly thrown knot.

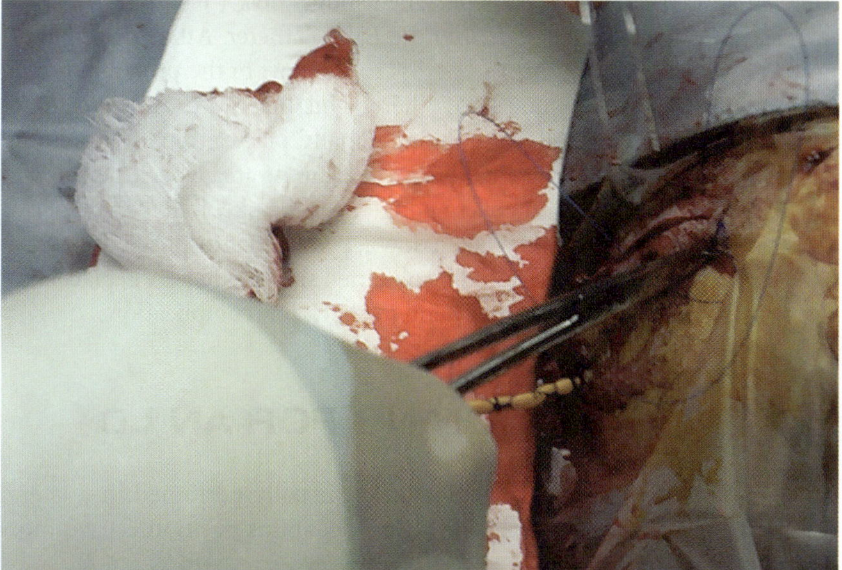

FIGURE 4.16. Suturing the incision. The suture is started at the top of the incision in a running fashion because a deep bite can be taken without threat to the catheter. As the suture is run, it is kept loose so that skin edges can be raised to visualize the galea and the catheter. After the last bite, the suture line is pulled tight and an instrumented tie is used to secure the suture line.

have observed some surgeons cutting the catheter at the puncture point and using a straight metal connector, we refrain from doing this because it breaks the sterility barrier of the antibiotic-coated catheter, which may come apart when the catheter is being removed if it is not attached snugly.

Final Steps

With the incision closed, secure the rest of the catheter. We place a BioPatch (Ethicon; Johnson & Johnson) around the exit point. We make a large loop around the incision and secure it to the skin using 2-0 nylon. Some surgeons prefer to use the suture collar, a soft white plastic tab in the EVD catheter kit. We find suture collar useful as the first anchor point after the catheter exits the skin. The needle is passed through the suture collar as close as possible to the catheter without puncturing it, then through skin with a substantial amount of slack. The suture collar is then tightly secured to the skin using square knots. At the other two anchor points, a loose stitch is thrown through the skin, the catheter is laid on the knot of the stitch, and snug knots are then made on top of the catheter, with care taken to avoid occluding it.

The assistant removes the proximal tubing from the previously prepared CSF collection chamber from its sterile bag and hands it off to the surgeon. Remove the red cap on the catheter. Then snugly tie a 4-0 silk suture where the clear plastic adapter inserts into the EVD catheter. After making multiple knots, bring the suture ends across to the port of the proximal tubing system and tie multiple snug knots there. This marries the EVD catheter with the proximal CSF collection tubing. Finally, place a thin layer of liquid adhesive (Mastisol, Eloquest Healthcare, Ltd.) in the area where the hair was shaved. Place a sterile drain cover sponge over the site, followed by perforated tape. The drapes are then taken down, and trash is disposed of safely. A head computed tomogram should be obtained shortly after EVD placement to confirm positioning of the EVD and to check for complications.

PATIENT POSITIONING FOR AN LD

Lumbar punctures and LD placements are usually perfomed in a lateral decubitus or a sitting position. The lateral decubitus position is used most often for LD insertion.

For the lateral decubitus position, the patient, if alert, is allowed to position himself or herself. The side that the patient faces depends on the layout of the room. The surgeon will want the most space on the side where the surgeon will be situated. The bed can be unlocked and pushed to provide more room on one side. When the patient is intubated, it is easier to turn the patient to the side of the ventilator. In either scenario, once the patient is turned onto one side, the back of the patient should be flush with the side of the bed. The knees and hips are flexed preliminarily. A pillow is often placed in between the patient's knees. If the head of the bed is elevated, it can be leveled. A chair is brought to this side for the surgeon. The surgeon elevates the bed to a level that will be comfortable while the surgeon is sitting.

Placing the patient in the sitting position can also be considered. This position is typically used with awake patients. The patient sits at the edge of the bed and moves backward to bend the knees right at the edge of the bed. This placement minimizes the distance the surgeon must reach. A personal table or Mayo stand is placed in front of the patient with a pillow on it. The patient then leans over and rests on the pillow on the table. A chair is obtained for the surgeon, and height of the bed is adjusted accordingly to allow a comfortable working angle for the surgeon. We have also used this arrangement with intubated patients. It is a multiperson coordinated task that can also be done to place the patient facing the ventilator. With the patient in the sitting position, the midline is much easier to identify, especially in obese patients. Placing the patient in a sitting position should be considered when it proves difficult to access the lumbar cistern with the patient in the lateral position as this has prevented trips to interventional radiology for placement on numerous occasions.

LD PROCEDURE: STEPS, NUANCES, AND COMPLICATION MANAGEMENT

Skin Preparation

Unlike an EVD, an LD rarely requires hair trimming in this region of the body. However, cleansing is important, and the entire lower back is given a round of washing and drying. Next, the insertion site is marked. A sterile marker is used to draw the Tuffier line, most likely marking the L4-L5 interspace. Knowledge of the midline is especially important. Superficial tissues can shift downward, especially with a large body habitus, which can give a false impression of the midline. We have gotten into the habit of drawing the spinous processes for at least 4 to 5 levels. The entry point is marked, and the marker point is pressed into the skin. The CSF collection chamber is prepared as noted above for the EVD. All equipment is opened, and the surgeon dons sterile dress. We prefer to start with an open-tipped lumbar catheter because it has the benefit of allowing obstructions to be flushed proximally into the thecal sac, if necessary. The skin is prepped with sterilizing solution in the same manner as for EVDs and allowed to dry. All markings are redrawn.

The sterile towels are placed in the same order each time. The first towel is placed between the bed and the patient, with an end of the towel folded over the fingers to prevent contamination with the unprepped skin. Then towels are placed across the lower back or buttocks and the lower thorax. Finally, the last towel is placed over the upper side of the patient (Fig. 4.17). The half drape is placed on the upper thorax. The last towel is placed on the side of the surgeon where the equipment table is located.

Just prior to incision, a surgical time-out is taken by all the medical personnel in the room to confirm that we have the correct patient, procedure, site, side, indications, allergies, and so forth. This double-checking process for LDs is the same as that for EVDs.

Skin Puncture

As for an EVD, we use an epinephrine-lidocaine 1:200,000 premixed solution. We create a superficial welt. Then we switch to a longer 21-gauge

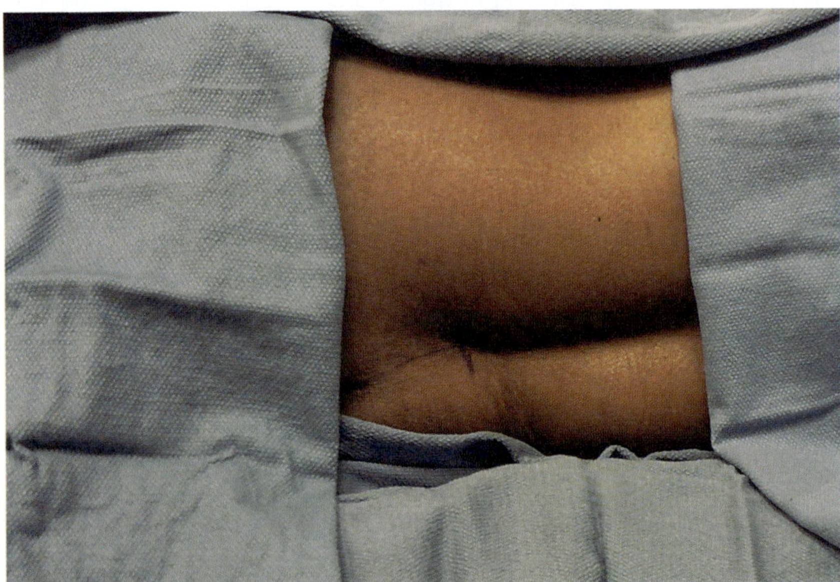

FIGURE 4.17. Draping for a lumbar drain. Sterile towels are placed in the same order every time after the sterilizing solution has dried. The lower towel with a fold over the fingers is placed first. The two side towels are placed next, followed by the top towel last.

intravenous needle and insert it to its full length. Spinal needles are typically 90 mm (about 3.5 inches) long, whereas this needle is 38 mm (1.5 inches). Regardless, we always draw back first to ensure that we haven't inadvertently entered the thecal sac. At the full length of the needle, you can typically palpate the spinous processes, and potentially the lamina, with the needle point. The periosteal space is particularly sensitive, and we direct most of the anesthetic here. We allow the anesthetic to work for 2 to 3 minutes. During this time, the assistant administers the perioperative antibiotics and any additional doses of sedative and analgesic medication. The manometer is assembled, and the instruments are laid out in their order of use (Fig. 4.18). The catheter is flushed once with sterile saline.

The next step is to insert the Tuohy needle at the area of the lidocaine welt. Insert it with the bevel pointed up the side of the patient (Fig. 4.19A). Direct it perpendicular to the skin and insert it at an even pace. You must have a mental map of the midline in mind while advancing the needle, with your target being the belly button of the patient. If an obstacle is encountered that prevents further advancement, the assistant can maximally flex the patient at the hips into the fetal position. The fetal position opens the interspinous space, allowing you to resume advancing the needle. If further advancement is still not possible, we prefer to "map" the area by lightly bouncing the tip of the needle on the bone. Most likely, you will encounter

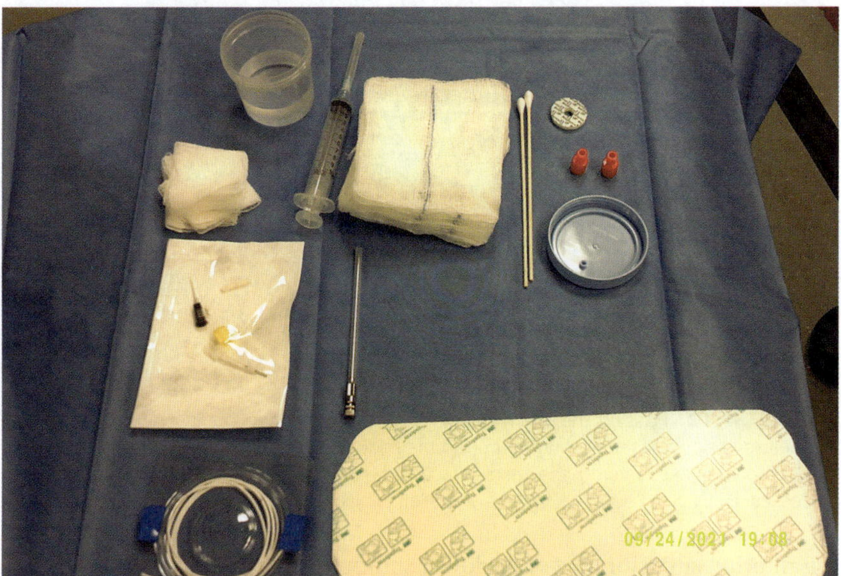

FIGURE 4.18. Lumbar drain kit. The kit equipment is inspected and laid out to ensure that everything needed is present.

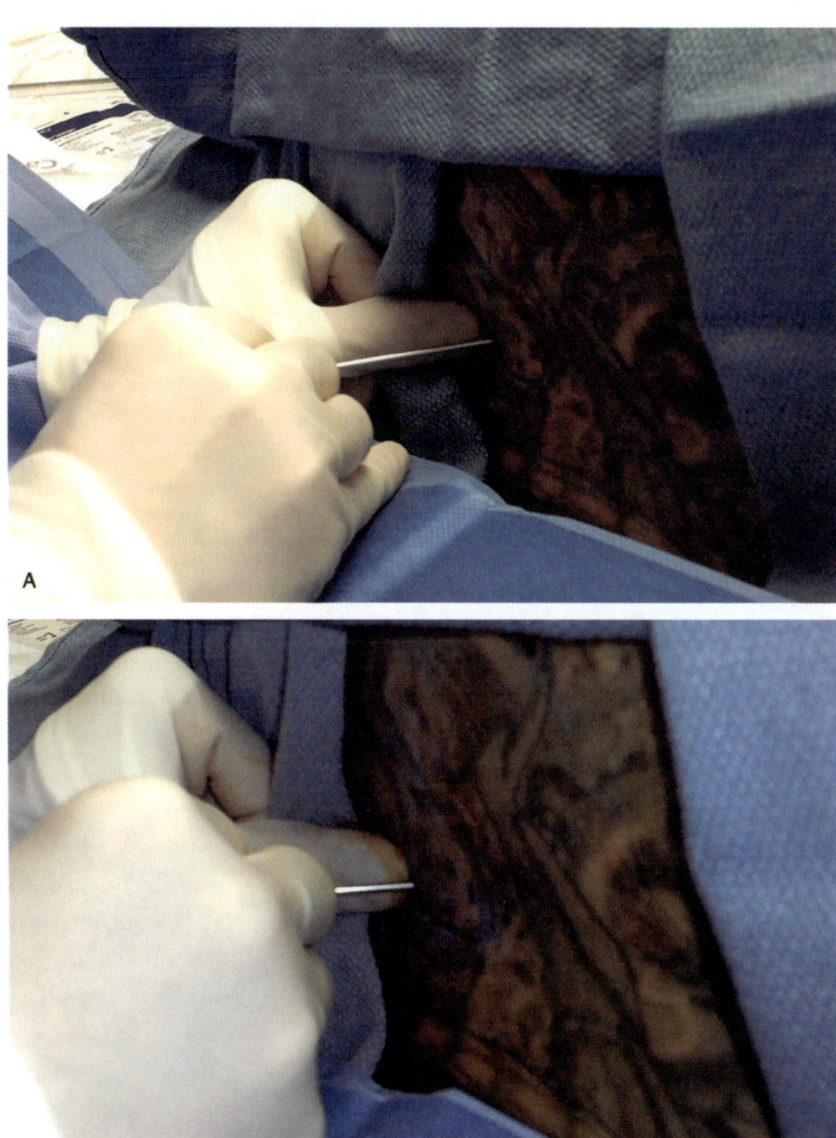

FIGURE 4.19. Passing the Tuohy needle. **A.** The Tuohy needle is inserted into the welt. The needle is slowly inserted, staying true to the midline at an angle pointing to the belly button. If difficulty is encountered, the needle tip can be used to "map out" the lamina and spinous processes. **B.** Once a "pop" is felt, the stylet is left in place until the catheter is prepared.

the anterior-superior part of the lower spinous process or one of its laminae. When this occurs, withdraw the needle halfway and change the angle to superior by lowering your hand toward your feet. If this change in angle is too steep, the needle will likely encounter the undersurface of the superior spinous process. Achieving access requires threading the needle through this space. Entrance into the thecal sac has been described as a popping sensation but that sensation is more likely produced by going through the ligamentum flavum (Fig. 4.19B). Once you feel this sensation, remove the stylet and check for CSF flow. As for an EVD, a minimal amount of CSF is released with an LD. The manometer can be attached to the needle at this point to record pressure, if necessary.

If you encounter an impassible bony obstacle at a superficial depth, then likely the entry point is above a spinous process rather than at the interspinous space. If CSF flow is present but sluggish, turn the needle so that the bevel faces toward the head of the patient. If the flow is still sluggish, advance the needle only after reinserting the stylet. If you advance the needle too deeply, you will encounter the posterior surface of the vertebral body. Slowly withdraw the needle and check the CSF flow. If you observe brisk bleeding after removing the stylet, you should replace the stylet. The paraspinal muscles have a rich vascular supply and injury with a 14-gauge Tuohy needle can cause bleeding that will subside without further intervention. Surgeons often fear that they will injure the aorta or vena cava. However, the great vessels are usually located at the depth of the mid-vertebral body; thus, reaching them with a regular Tuohy needle is impossible in most cases. We have found no documented evidence of this type of injury in the neurosurgery literature. In contrast, injury to the spinal nerve roots can happen and has been reported to occur with 25-gauge needles although injury from a larger Tuohy needle is less likely.[5] Injury to the conus at the L3-L4 and L4-L5 levels is extremely unlikely, as discussed previously.

Passing the Catheter

After the needle is in a satisfactory location, you can insert the catheter. The catheter has a black mark that indicates it has been inserted the full length of the needle (Fig. 4.20). The catheter is quickly loaded into the needle shaft to prevent CSF egress. If the catheter proceeds easily after this point, then it should be continued at least to the 15-cm mark.

If resistance is encountered, the catheter will require troubleshooting. If the catheter has passed the point marking the full length of the needle, you should not attempt to withdraw it. Doing so may cause the catheter to fracture into the lumbar cistern. A common cause of resistance is an angle of entry that is too steep, thereby causing the catheter to run into canal walls or spinal nerve roots. You can rectify this problem by turning

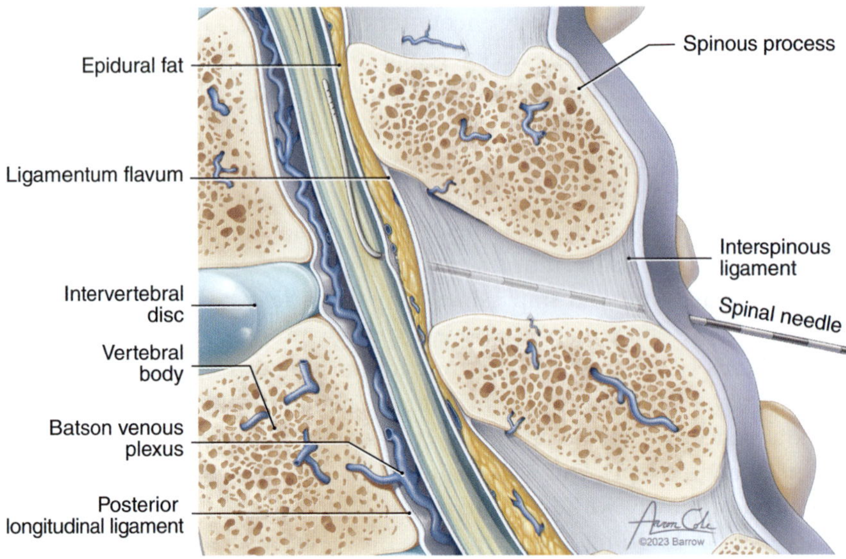

FIGURE 4.20. Artist's illustration demonstrating the lumbar catheter entering the cerebro-spinal fluid space. The catheter should easily pass cranially between the nerve roots.

the bevel toward the head, if this has not already been done, and by lowering your hand toward your feet. You can also rotate the catheter while advancing it. In the same motion, you can slightly withdraw the needle. If the catheter has not passed this mark and none of these maneuvers is successful, withdraw it and try a closed-tip LD catheter with a stylet. The stylet gives the catheter extra rigidity. Once the stylet is past the 15-cm mark, remove it by pulling on it while holding the needle and catheter in place. If this maneuver is also not successful, the entire catheter and the Tuohy needle should be removed, and an attempt at LD placement should be made at a different level.

Final Steps

After the catheter is in position, drop it below the level of the patient to confirm CSF flow. Once flow is confirmed, remove the Tuohy needle. Feed the catheter forward with one hand while pulling back on the needle shaft with the other. When the needle is out of the skin, work it back along the catheter, while continuing to hold the catheter in a fixed position against the skin. Then ensure CSF flow (Fig. 4.21). With the needle completely off, place a clear plastic adapter on the catheter, followed by a yellow cap. If the catheter is inadvertently pulled during this process, you must assess how much catheter remains inside the patient. Ideally, the catheter should be at

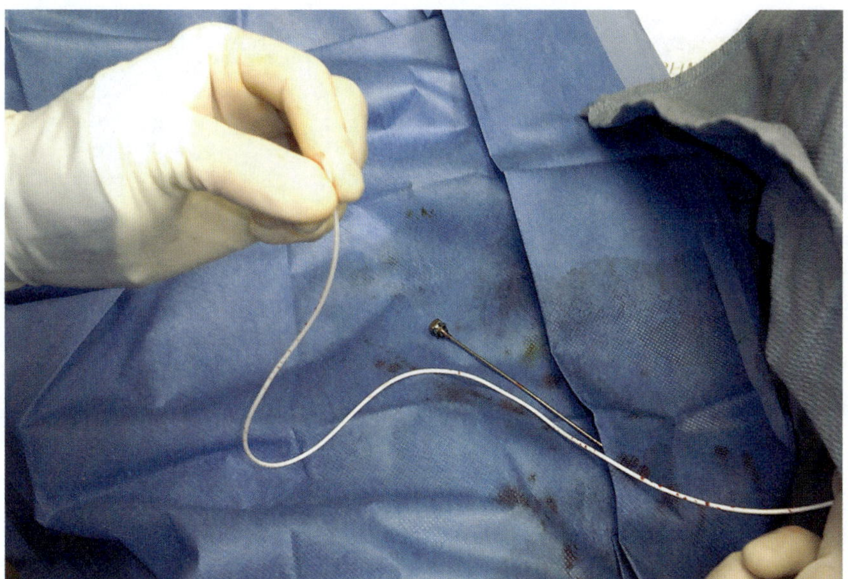

FIGURE 4.21. Checking cerebrospinal fluid (CSF) flow. After the stylet is removed, CSF flow is confirmed.

the 15-cm mark or greater. We suggest removal and replacement at 7.5 cm or less.

Instead of securing the drain at the exit point, some may use a tunneling technique to place the lumbar catheter. This step may be applied in cases where CSF drainage will be needed for prolonged periods of time. While we do not have experience with this method, Hahn and colleagues[6] have written an excellent technical note describing the technique.

As when placing an EVD, the catheter for an LD is secured to the skin at its exit point. Given the much smaller diameter of the LD catheter, 2-0 nylon suture will not give the same grip as in an EVD procedure, so we recommend using 4-0 nylon suture instead. This step can also be performed using a purse-string technique, with the tails of the suture crossed over onto the catheter and knotted multiple times. This knotting technique requires more precision than that needed for the EVD catheter, because the LD catheter is easier to occlude. After placing the suture, confirm CSF flow. If you cannot restore flow with the suture in place, remove it and use a suture collar instead. If the LD catheter is still occluded, it may require flushing and priming. Attach a syringe with sterile normal saline and lightly aspirate it if necessary, infusing less than 1 mL saline proximally.

Finally, a BioPatch should be placed over the exit site. Attach the LD catheter in a sterile fashion to the CSF collection chamber proximal tube.

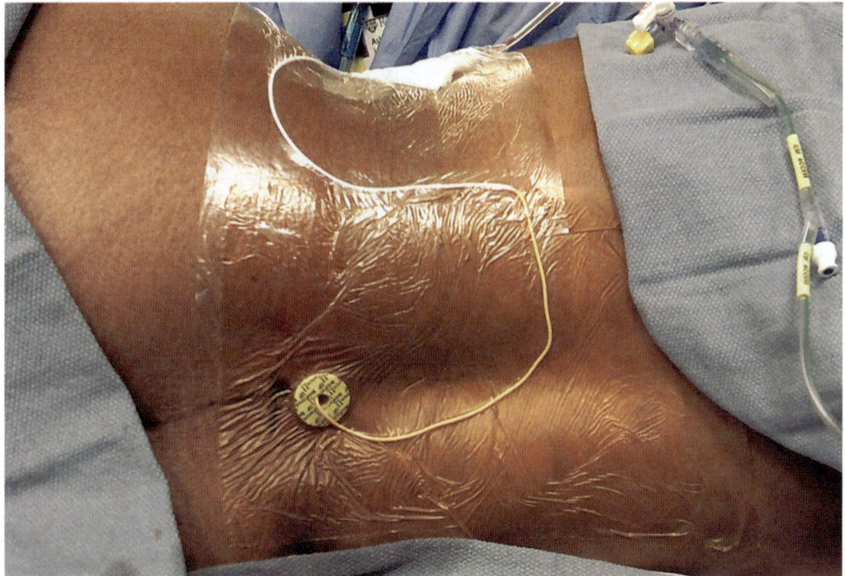

FIGURE 4.22. Lumbar drain dressing. After the drain is secured at its exit point, a BioPatch is placed, then an Ioban dressing is placed.

As with an EVD, use a 4-0 silk suture to secure the LD catheter to the clear plastic adapter, then cross the suture over to the CSF collection chamber proximal tubing adapter and tie it. Loop the lumbar catheter around the exit site. Place a sheet of Ioban (3M) so that no air bubbles are present on the skin. The Ioban acts as an occlusive dressing, covering the skin from above the buttocks to the lower thorax and to each flank. Bring the catheter to one side and secure it with tape. When the procedure is finished, the drapes are taken down, and medical waste is safely disposed (Fig. 4.22).

ABBREVIATIONS

CSF, cerebrospinal fluid

EVD, external ventricular drain

LD, lumbar drain

REFERENCES

1. Dumville JC, McFarlane E, Edwards P, Lipp A, Holmes A, Liu Z. Preoperative skin antiseptics for preventing surgical wound infections after clean surgery. *Cochrane Database Syst Rev*. 2015;(4):CD003949. doi:10.1002/14651858.CD003949.pub4.
2. Tolcher MC, Whitham MD, El-Nashar SA, Clark SL. Chlorhexidine-alcohol compared with povidone-iodine preoperative skin antisepsis for cesarean delivery: a systematic review and meta-analysis. *Am J Perinatol*. 2019;36(2):118-123. doi:10.1055/s-0038-1669907.
3. Liu S, Carpenter RL, Chiu AA, McGill TJ, Mantell SA. Epinephrine prolongs duration of subcutaneous infiltration of local anesthesia in a dose-related manner: correlation with magnitude of vasoconstriction. *Reg Anesth*. 1995;20(5):378-384.
4. Amoo M, Henry J, Javadpour M. Common trajectories for freehand frontal ventriculostomy: a systematic review. *World Neurosurg*. 2021;146:292-297. doi:10.1016/j.wneu.2020.11.065.
5. Reina MA, Lopez A, Villanueva MC, De Andres JA, Martin S. [Possibility of cauda equina nerve root damage from lumbar punctures performed with 25-gauge Quincke and Whitacre needles]. *Rev Esp Anestesiol Reanim*. 2005;52(5):267-275. Posibilidad de lesion en las raices nerviosas de la cola de caballo en relacion con las punciones lumbares realizadas con agujas 25-G Quincke y Whitacre.
6. Hahn M, Murali R, Couldwell WT. Tunneled lumbar drain. Technical note. *J Neurosurg*. 2002;96(6):1130-1131. doi:10.3171/jns.2002.96.6.1130.

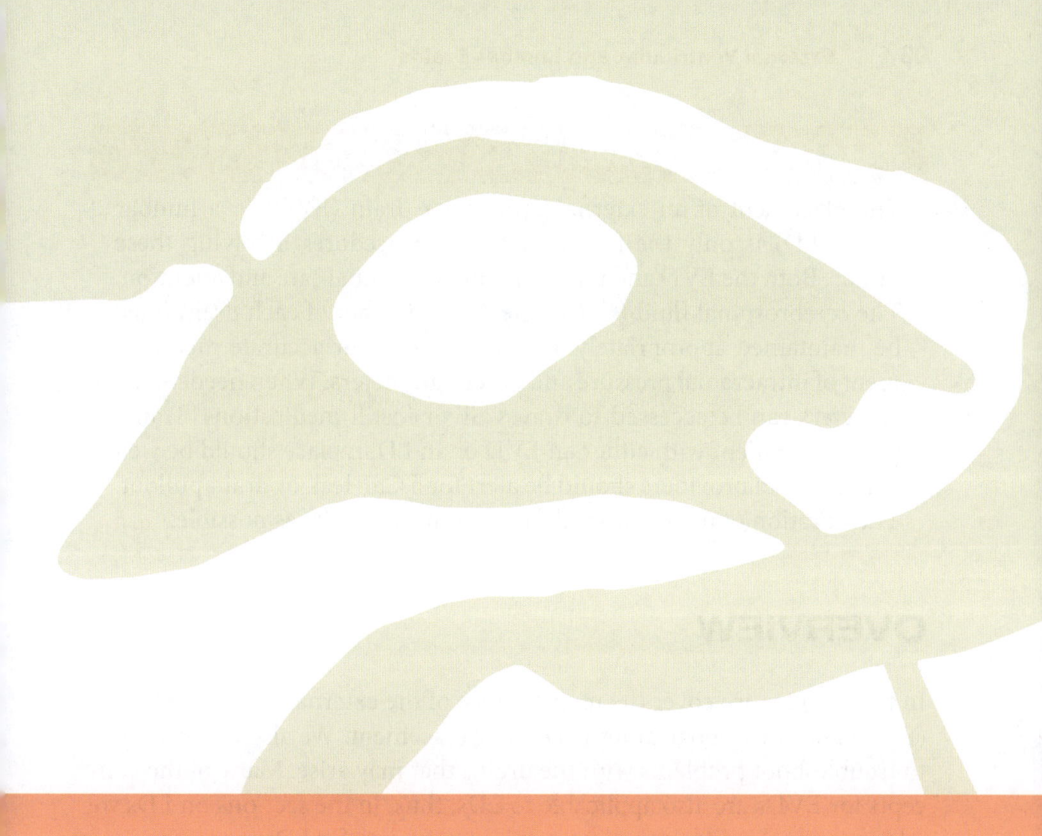

CHAPTER 5

Postplacement Care

CHAPTER SUMMARY

The placement of an external ventricular drain (EVD) or a lumbar drain (LD) is only the first part of the procedures involving these drains. Both the EVD and the LD require continual care and attention. The cerebrospinal fluid (CSF) collection chamber of each drain must be maintained appropriately. Doing so allows for accurate measurement of intracranial pressure and other parameters. When needed, the catheters can be accessed to draw CSF or instill medications. Transporting a patient with either an EVD or an LD in place should be well planned, and providers should be alert for a CSF leak or drain pullout. The duration of use of either drain should be as brief as possible.

OVERVIEW

In this chapter, we cover the maintenance of the external ventricular drain (EVD) and the lumbar drain (LD) after placement. We also describe how to troubleshoot problems with the drains that may arise. Many of the concepts for EVDs are also applicable to LDs; thus, in the sections on LDs we address only the differences in postplacement care for LDs.

EVD MAINTENANCE

Dressing

After the EVD has been placed, but before the sterile drapes are taken down, a dressing is placed over the site of the drain. Practices vary with regard to the type of dressing and how often it should be changed. Some authors recommend an occlusive dressing, whereas others recommend a nonocclusive dressing. A randomized controlled trial showed that dressings containing chlorhexidine reduced subcutaneous colonization of EVDs.[1]

Although consensus statements have not given definitive recommendations for EVD dressing, we suggest using a BioPatch (Ethicon; Johnson & Johnson) at the drain exit point. The fine hair that remains on the skin after clipping makes an occlusive dressing difficult to maintain. We prefer a sterile gauze drain sponge (Fig. 5.1). Neuroscience nursing assessment is performed at least every 2 to 4 hours to ensure that the sponge has not become saturated with cerebrospinal fluid (CSF). The dressing should be changed every 3 days or whenever it becomes soiled or dislodged. The

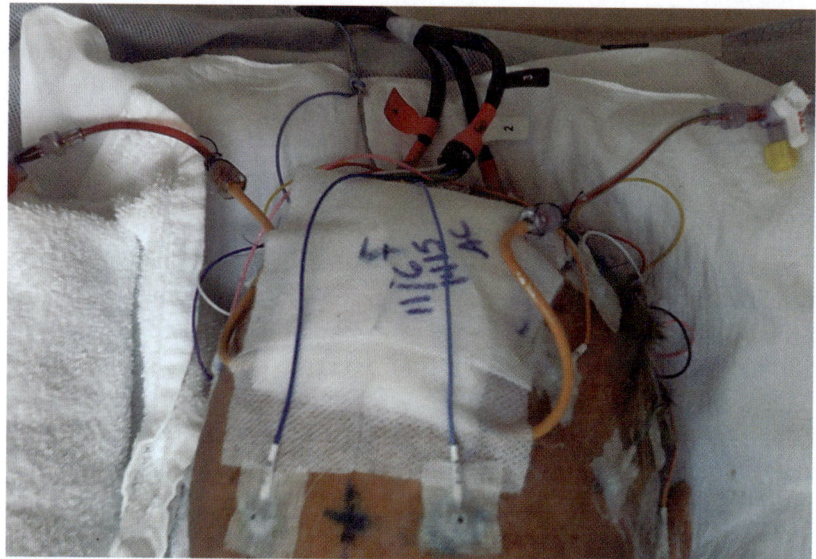

FIGURE 5.1. External ventricular drain (EVD) dressing. The types of dressing used at our institutions for EVDs are a BioPatch covered by a sterile gauze dressing taped on all four sides. To facilitate an appropriate changing schedule, we write the date the dressing was placed and the name of the provider who placed it on the dressing itself. This dressing also helps to mark the boundaries for where electroencephalogram electrodes can be placed on the scalp.

BioPatch dressing is replaced at least every 7 days. Replacement should be performed in a sterile manner using sterile gloves and sterile sponges. Hair around the area of the drain should be kept short (but not shaved) until the drain is removed.

CSF Collection Chamber

Numerous CSF collection chambers are available, including the Codman EDS 3, the Integra AccuDrain, and the Medtronic Becker system. The collection chamber can be prepared by the surgeon's assistant or a neuroscience nurse while the drain is being placed. The drainage system is attached to an intravenous pole, with care taken to keep the proximal tubing sterile (Fig. 5.2A). A CSF pressure transducer as well as sterile red caps and sterile syringes filled with preservative-free normal saline are opened onto a sterile field. Sterile gloves are worn to attach the transducer to the CSF collection system at the zero point on the stopcock. The tubing of the transducer is removed. A syringe is attached to this hub. The stopcock is turned, the transducer is flushed, and then a red cap is placed at the end of the pressure transducer (Fig. 5.2B). The three-way stopcock to the Buretrol (ie, the fluid volume limiter) is turned off, and the system is flushed proximally until fluid emanates from the end of the proximal tubing (Fig. 5.2C). The stopcock is turned again, and the system is flushed distally into the Buretrol (Fig. 5.2D). Finally, the stopcock is turned one final time, off to the transducer. The syringe is removed (Fig. 5.2E). At this point, the transducer wire is connected to the monitor and the drain is zeroed by pressing the appropriate "zero" button on the monitor. Once the preparation of the collection chamber is complete, a red cap is placed on the hub (Figs. 5.2F and 5.2G).

When the surgeon is ready, the proximal tubing is handed off in a sterile manner and the three-way stopcock at the zero point is turned off to the Buretrol. The collection system is set so that the zero point is level with the tragus of the patient (Fig. 5.3). The zero point is aligned with the tragus using the carpenter level or laser pointer in the EVD kit. Next, the draining pressure is set by moving the arm where the Buretrol is attached either up or down. The draining pressure is based on the clinical situation.

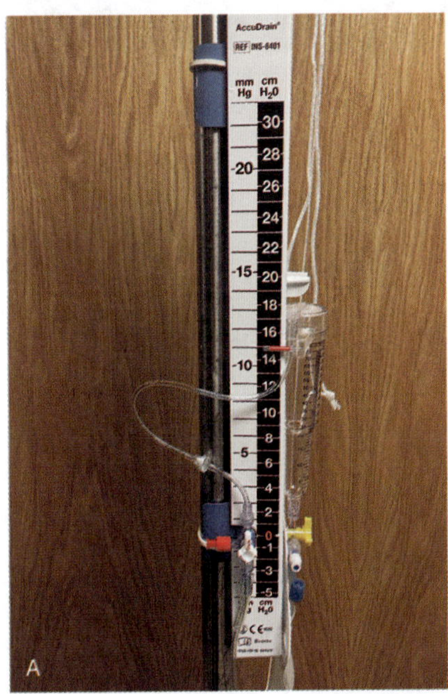

FIGURE 5.2. Cerebrospinal fluid (CSF) collection system setup. **A.** The CSF collection chamber is attached to a pole. **B.** The pressure transducer is attached *(red arrowhead),* the stopcock is turned off to the system, and a sterile saline syringe is attached to flush the transducer. **C.** The transducer stopcock is turned off to the transducer, and the CSF collection chamber three-way stopcock *(red arrowhead)* to the Buretrol is turned off, which allows the proximal system line to be flushed. **D.** The system three-way stopcock *(red arrowhead)* is turned off to the proximal line so that the Buretrol line can be flushed. **E.** The syringe is removed, and the transducer stopcock *(red arrowhead)* is turned off to the system so that it can be zeroed. **F.** All stopcocks in the system *(red arrowheads)* are placed in the intracranial pressure–transducing mode (ie, clamped). **G.** The system with all stopcocks *(red arrowhead)* in the drain mode.

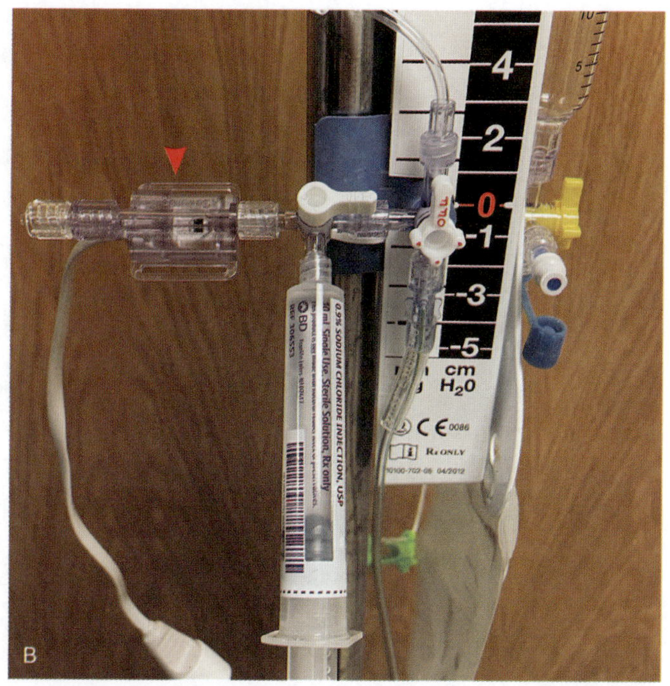

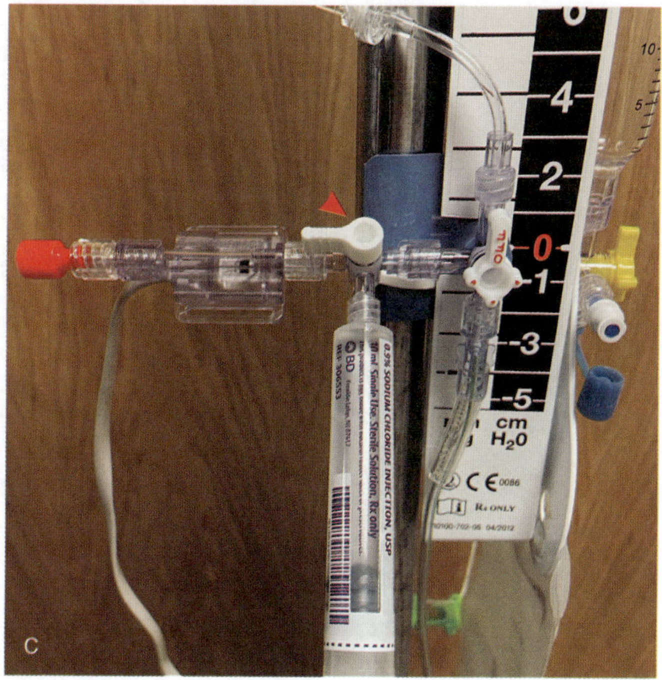

FIGURE 5.2. (Continued)

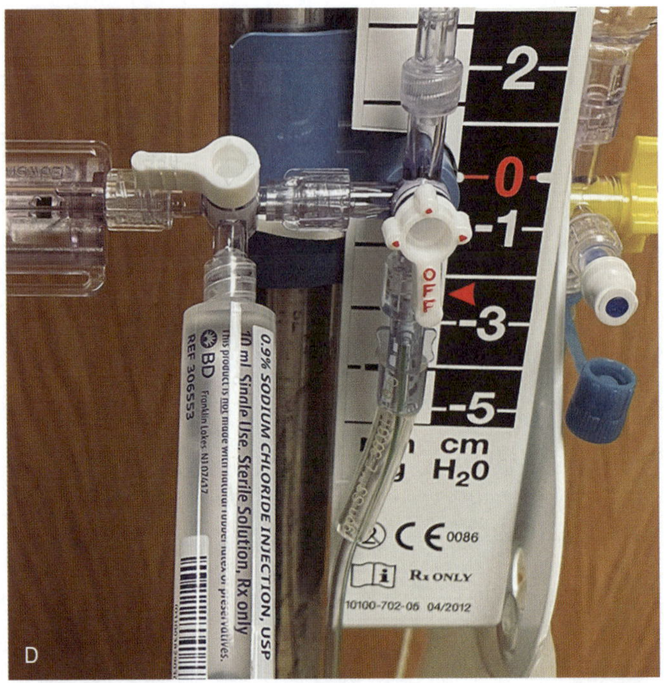

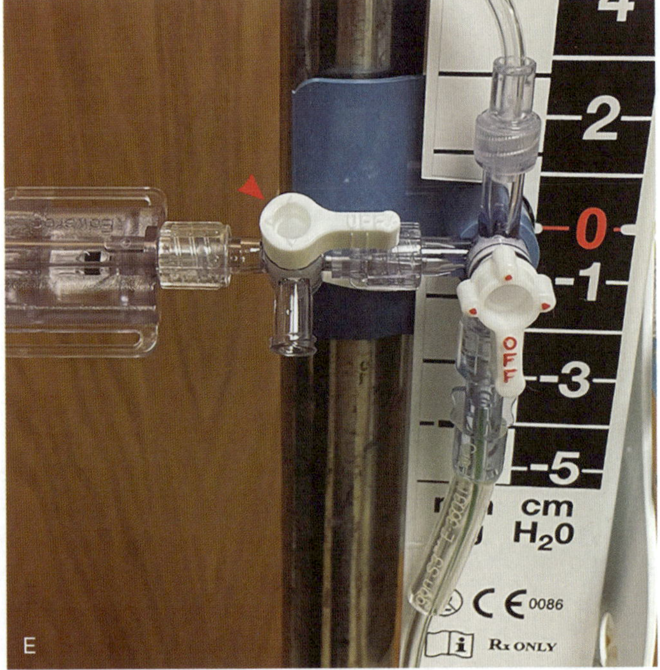

FIGURE 5.2. (Continued)

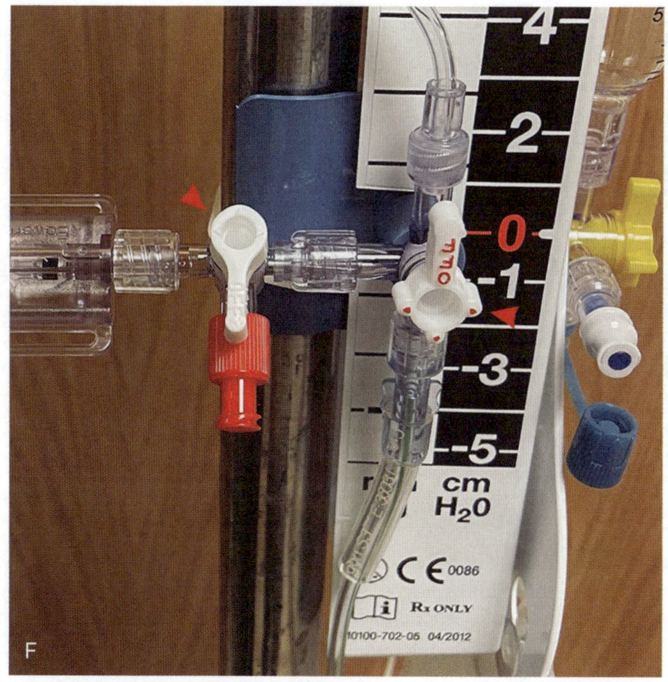

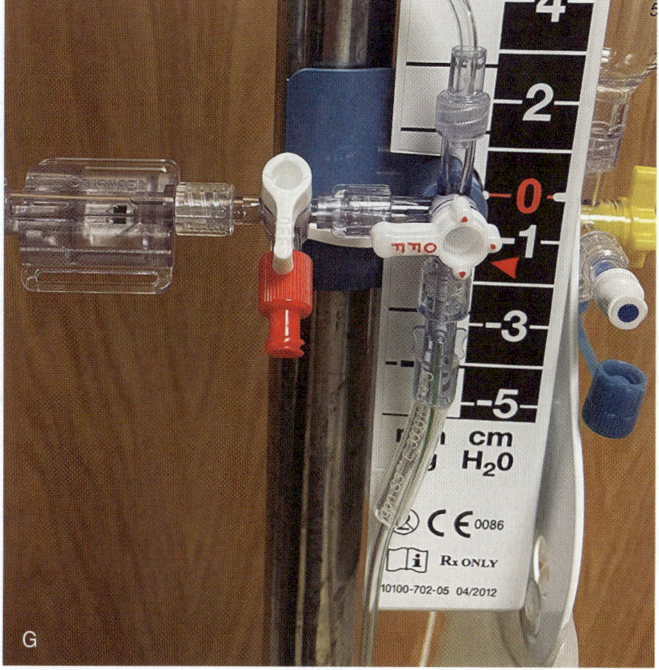

FIGURE 5.2. (Continued)

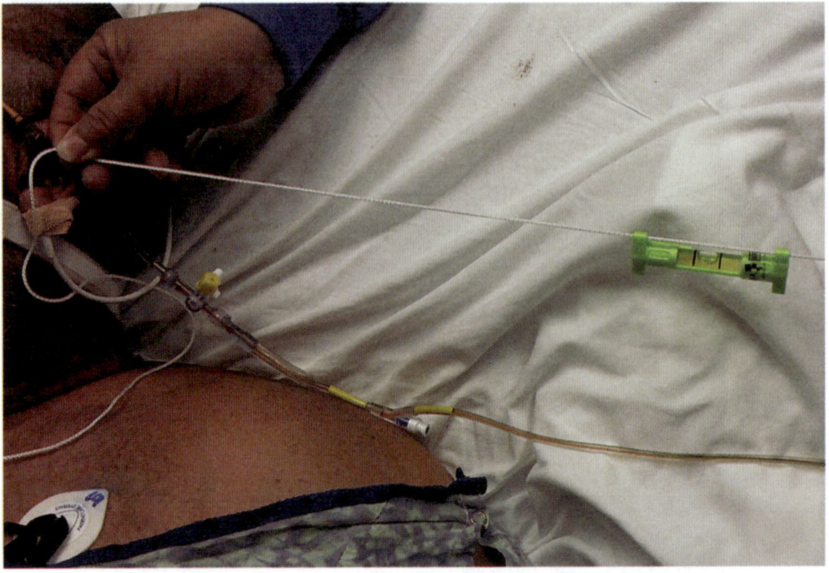

FIGURE 5.3. Leveling to the tragus. The external ventricular drain (EVD) is leveled to the tragus of the ear using either a laser pointer or a carpenter level, depending on which is included in the EVD kit used at your institution.

For patients with mass lesions or traumatic brain injury and high intracranial pressure (ICP), the draining pressure can be set as low as zero or 5 cm H_2O. For patients with untreated aneurysms, it is typically set at 15 or 20 cm H_2O. The drainage pattern can be continuous, with intermittent clamping of the drain to transduce an ICP or with clamping at all times to transduce ICP and with an intermittent opening to drain CSF. We do not recommend leaving the stopcock in a position for both ICP transduction and CSF draining because this position may not allow accurate ICP measurement. The collection chamber should be assessed at least every 2 to 4 hours to ensure that it is functioning properly and that the stopcock is in the appropriate position. Any number of wires, monitors, and tubing around the patient have been known to catch a corner of the stopcock and turn it to the wrong setting.

Other CSF collection chambers, such as the LimiTorr and MoniTorr (Integra LifeSciences Corp.), have traditionally been used only with LDs. These chambers are limited regarding how much CSF they can drain, which theoretically should prevent overdrainage of CSF. However, many providers are not comfortable relying on this mechanism for protection, and in 2019 the LimiTorr and MoniTorr chambers underwent a class 1 device recall by the U.S. Food and Drug Administration for potential breakage of a stopcock on each device (https://www.accessdata.fda.gov/scripts/cdrh/cfdocs/cfRes/res.cfm?ID=172227).

If any part of the CSF collection chamber is believed to be contaminated, the best practice is to completely change out the entire collection system. A clamp is placed on the EVD catheter before doing so to prevent the release of CSF when detaching the collection chamber. All replacement equipment should be opened in a sterile fashion, primed as described earlier, and attached in a sterile fashion. Routine changes of the collection system should not be performed.[2]

The collection chamber should be kept upright at all times and emptied into the collection bag when nearly full. Some systems have a filter paper on the top of the Buretrol, which helps maintain suction within the chamber as it is raised or lowered. When this filter paper becomes damp or is damaged, suction may no longer work.

ICP, Cerebral Perfusion Pressure, and Waveforms

ICP values will be generated when the stopcock diverts the entire CSF column to the transducer. For ICP monitoring indications, see Chap. 1. Cerebral perfusion pressure (CPP) can be calculated as mean arterial pressure (MAP) derived from an arterial line minus ICP:

$$CPP = MAP - ICP$$

In a recent consensus statement on severe traumatic brain injury, a four-tiered system was proposed for management of ICP.[3] Table 5.1 summarizes these management guidelines and their levels of evidence from the most recent Brain Trauma Foundation guidelines.[3-5] Although these recommendations are intended for patients with traumatic brain injury, most are applicable to almost all patients with increased ICP.

There has been discussion about how best to use the waveform to monitor ICP in patients with EVDs and LDs. With each cardiac cycle, there is a transient increase and decrease in the volume of blood within the blood vessels of the brain. These changes generate a triphasic peak waveform: P1 (systolic peak or percussion wave), P2 (tidal wave), and P3 (venous return or dicrotic wave) (Fig. 5.4).[6] In a patient with a less compliant brain, P2 has been described as increasing in amplitude. Kirkness et al[7] published an excellent summary of these physiologic changes and how they manifest (Table 5.2). Additionally, Lundberg waves, which occur over a much longer period (minutes to hours), herald an increase in ICP. Volume pressure tests, pulse pressure analysis, and reactivity indices are becoming increasingly common to determine the elastance of the brain and where it stands on the compliance curve of the Monro-Kellie doctrine.[6] These indices, when combined with multimodal monitoring technology, such as the Micromed

TABLE 5.1: LEVELS OF EVIDENCE FOR TIERED MANAGEMENT OF ELEVATED INTRACRANIAL PRESSURE*

Tier/Intervention	Evidence Level	Notes on Treatment Recommendations
Tier 0		
Admit to intensive care unit		
Conduct serial evaluation of neurologic status and pupillary function		
Elevate head of bed to 30-45°		
Administer analgesia for pain		
Implement endotracheal intubation and mechanical ventilation	IIB	
Maintain $SpO_2 \geq 94\%$		
Monitor end-tidal CO_2		
Sedate for agitation of ventilator synchrony		
Manage temperature (treat if core temp above 38°C)		

Monitor ICP	IIB	Treat ICP >22 mm Hg because values above this level are associated with increased mortality. Manage severe TBI using ICP monitoring to reduce in-hospital and 2-week postinjury mortality. Monitor ICP in all salvageable TBI patients (GCS score 3-8 after resuscitation) with an abnormal CT revealing hematomas, contusions, swelling, herniation, or compressed basal cisterns. ICP monitoring is indicated in patients with severe TBI and a normal CT with $\geq$2 of these criteria at admission: age >40 years, unilateral or bilateral motor posturing, and SBP <90 mm Hg.
Maintain CPP $\geq$60 mm Hg	IIB	Manage severe TBI patients using guidelines-based recommendations for CPP monitoring to decrease 2-week mortality. Target CPP value is 60-70 mm Hg for survival and favorable outcomes. The minimum optimal CPP threshold is unclear and may depend on the autoregulatory status of the patient.
Conduct advanced cerebral monitoring	III	Conduct jugular bulb monitoring of $AVDO_2$, to inform management decisions, as it may reduce mortality and improve outcomes at 3 and 6 months postinjury. Avoid jugular venous saturation <50% to reduce mortality and improve outcome.
Maintain hemoglobin $\geq$7 g/dL		
Avoid hyponatremia		
Optimize venous outflow from the head		

TABLE 5.1: LEVELS OF EVIDENCE FOR TIERED MANAGEMENT OF ELEVATED INTRACRANIAL PRESSURE* (Continued)

Tier/Intervention	Evidence Level	Notes on Treatment Recommendations
Insert arterial line	III	Maintain SBP $\geq$100 mm Hg for patients 50-69 years old or SBP $\geq$110 mm Hg for patients 15-49 or $\geq$70 years old to decrease mortality and improve outcomes.
Consider central line		
Consider antiepileptics for 1 week	IIA	Avoid prophylactic use of phenytoin or valproate to prevent late PTS. Use phenytoin to decrease incidence of early PTS ($\leq$7 days of injury), when overall benefit outweighs associated complications. However, early PTS has not been associated with worse outcomes. Current evidence on efficacy and toxicity are insufficient to recommend levetiracetam over phenytoin to prevent early PTS.
Avoid corticosteroids	I	Avoid use of corticosteroids for reducing ICP or improving outcome. High-dose methylprednisolone is associated with increased mortality in patients with severe TBI and is contraindicated.
Start nutrition	IIA IIB	Feed patients to attain basal caloric replacement at least by day 5 and at most by day 7 postinjury to decrease mortality. Conduct transgastric jejunal feeding to reduce incidence of ventilator-associated pneumonia.
Tier 1		
Maintain CPP 60-70 mm Hg	III	Avoid aggressive attempts to maintain CPP >70 mm Hg with fluids and pressors because of risk of adult respiratory failure.
Increase analgesia to reduce ICP	IIB	

Increase sedation to reduce ICP	IIB	Avoid or use high-dose propofol with caution for control of ICP, as it can produce significant morbidity. Propofol is not considered to improve mortality or 6-month outcomes.
Maintain $PaCO_2$ at low-normal end (35-38 mm Hg/4.7-5.1 kPa)	IIB	Avoid prolonged prophylactic hyperventilation with $PaCO_2$ ≤25 mm Hg. Avoid hyperventilation during first 24 hours after injury when CBF is often critically reduced. Use hyperventilation as a temporizing measure to reduce elevated ICP. With hyperventilation, do not use $SjvO_2$ and $BtpO_2$ measurements to monitor oxygen delivery.
Administer mannitol by intermittent bolus (0.25-1.0 g/kg)	Evidence does not meet current standards[†]	Avoid arterial hypotension (SBP <90 mm Hg). Restrict mannitol use prior to ICP monitoring to only those patients with signs of transtentorial herniation or progressive neurologic deterioration not attributable to extracranial causes.
Administer hypertonic saline by intermittent bolus	Evidence does not meet current standards[†]	
Drain CSF if EVD in place; otherwise, place EVD only if ICP is monitored[‡]	III	Consider an EVD system zeroed at the midbrain for continuous rather than intermittent drainage of CSF to reduce the ICP burden more effectively. Use CSF drainage to lower ICP in patients with an initial GCS ≤8. Consider using antimicrobial-coated catheters to prevent catheter-related infections during CSF drainage.
Consider EEG monitoring		
Tier 2		
Monitor for mild hypocapnia (range 32-35 mm Hg/4.3-4.6 kPa)		

TABLE 5.1: LEVELS OF EVIDENCE FOR TIERED MANAGEMENT OF ELEVATED INTRACRANIAL PRESSURE* *(Continued)*

Tier/Intervention	Evidence Level	Notes on Treatment Recommendations
Evaluate for neuromuscular paralysis		
Conduct MAP challenge to assess cerebral autoregulation		
Raise CPP with boluses, vasopressors, or inotropes		
Tier 3		
Induce pentobarbital or thiopental coma, with dose titrated to ICP	IIB	Avoid administration of barbiturates to induce burst suppression measured by EEG as prophylaxis for intracranial hypertension. Use high-dose barbiturates to control elevated ICP refractory to maximum standard medical and surgical treatment while maintaining hemodynamic stability.

| Conduct decompressive craniectomy | IIA | Perform secondary DC for late refractory ICP elevation to reduce mortality and improve favorable outcomes. Secondary DC performed for early refractory ICP elevation does not improve mortality and favorable outcomes. Use a large frontotemporoparietal DC (not less than 12×15 cm or 15 cm in diameter) instead of a small frontotemporoparietal DC for reduced mortality and improved neurologic outcomes in patients with severe TBI. Perform secondary DC as a treatment for either early or late refractory ICP elevation to reduce ICP and duration of intensive care, although the effects and favorability of outcomes are uncertain. |
| Induce mild hypothermia (35-36°C) | IIB | Avoid early ($\leq$2.5 hours) and short-term ($\geq$48 hours postinjury) prophylactic hypothermia for patients with diffuse injury. |

$AVDO_2$, arteriovenous oxygen content difference; $BtpO_2$, brain tissue partial pressure of oxygen; CBF, cerebral blood flow; CO_2, carbon dioxide; CPP, cerebral perfusion pressure; CSF, cerebrospinal fluid; CT, computed tomogram; DC, decompressive craniectomy; EEG, electroencephalogram; EVD, external ventricular drain; GCS, Glasgow Coma Scale; ICP, intracranial pressure; MAP, mean arterial pressure; PaO_2, partial pressure of oxygen; PTS, posttraumatic seizures; SBP, systolic blood pressure; $SjvO_2$, jugular venous oxygen saturation; SpO_2, oxygen saturation; TBI, traumatic brain injury.

*Data from Hawryluk et al, 2019, Carney et al, 2017, and Hawryluk et al, 2020.[3-5]

†Recommendations from the previous edition (3rd ed.) of *Brain Trauma Foundation Guidelines* are not supported by evidence that meets current standards.

‡Although guidelines and consensus statements focus on EVDs for patients with TBI, evidence is minimal regarding which drainage system is superior and whether EVDs benefit patients with elevated ICP without TBI. Please refer to previous chapters for information on the use of lumbar drains in patients with nonobstructive hydrocephalus or a lack of mass effect or midline shift. Despite only level III evidence on antibiotic-coated catheters per the guidelines, we strongly recommend their use only.

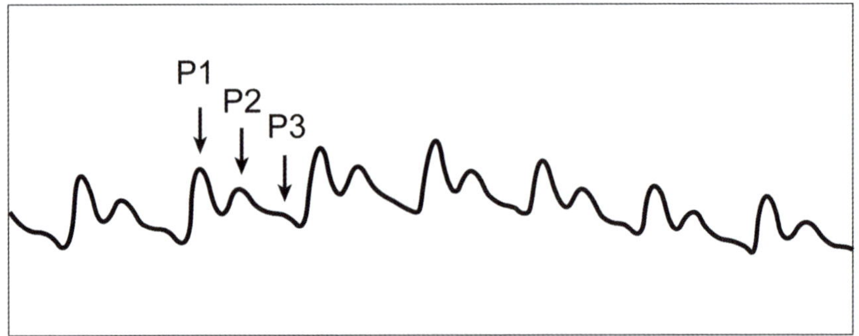

FIGURE 5.4. Intracranial pressure (ICP) waveforms. This figure shows the classic triphasic ICP waveform of P1, P2, and P3. Traditionally, P1 is called the percussion wave, P2 the tidal wave, and P3 the dicrotic wave. *Used with permission from Kirkness CJ, Mitchell PH, Burr RL, March KS, Newell DW. Intracranial pressure waveform analysis: clinical and research implications.* J Neurosci Nurs. *2000;32(5):271-277.*

TABLE 5.2: PHYSIOLOGIC CHANGES AND THEIR MANIFESTATION ON INTRACRANIAL PRESSURE WAVEFORMS

Condition	ICP and Waveform Changes
Rapidly expanding mass lesion	Increased mean ICP Increased ICP waveform amplitude
Increased or decreased CSF volume	Increased or decreased mean ICP Increased or decreased ICP waveform amplitude Minimally changed ICP waveform configuration
Severe arterial hypotension	Decreased mean ICP Decreased ICP waveform amplitude, especially P1
Severe arterial hypertension	Increased mean ICP Increased ICP waveform amplitude
Severe hypercapnia and hypoxia	Increased mean ICP Increased ICP waveform amplitude Rounded ICP waveform due to increase in later waveform components
Hyperventilation	Decreased mean ICP Decreased ICP waveform amplitude P2, and to a lesser degree P3, with little change in P1
Jugular vein compression	Increased mean ICP Increased ICP waveform amplitude, mainly P2 and P3

CSF, cerebrospinal fluid; ICP, intracranial pressure; P1, systolic peak or percussion wave; P2, tidal wave; P3, venous return or dicrotic wave.

Used with permission from Kirkness et al, 2000.[7]

Moberg central nervous system monitor, hold promise for therapeutic intervention and improvement of patient outcomes.

Perhaps the more important consideration is the loss of a waveform that existed before placement of the EVD or LD. Any such loss should be investigated because the ICP values can no longer be guaranteed to be accurate in this situation. The entire EVD line should be inspected, from the catheter exit point to the Buretrol. Kinks around sutures or various other lines are often to blame. Debris or blood clotting can cause an occlusion. The stopcock should be checked to ensure that it is in the appropriate position, and the monitor should be checked to ensure that it is still attached. The monitor should be rezeroed, and the scale should be checked to ensure it is set appropriately. The Buretrol or the collection chamber can be lowered toward the floor. Either approach can create enough pressure differential between the two points to help clear an occlusion or to move CSF past a narrowing. Alternatively, the obstruction may require accessing the line and flushing it as discussed below.

If the ventricle is collapsed around the catheter or the choroid plexus has become entwined within the catheter holes, it can cause a functional obstruction resulting in the loss of waveform. If either condition is suspected or confirmed by imaging, the opposite maneuver to clearing an obstruction is required. In this case, the EVD can be clamped for a longer period to allow CSF to build up within the ventricle. If doing so facilitates drainage again, then a higher drainage pressure or a lower hourly rate of CSF drainage should be sought.

CSF Sampling and EVD Access

When intraventricular medication must be administered, CSF is being sampled, or an obstruction requires investigation, the clinician must access the EVD line. How frequently the system can be safely accessed is debatable. To date, no prospective randomized trials have addressed this concern; thus, recommendations are based on retrospective reviews. The argument for frequent and routine sampling of CSF is to isolate an infection before it worsens or appears clinically. Because cultures typically require 2 to 3 days for growth, the advantage of frequent sampling may be lost. Gram stain results can be obtained much more quickly but have been reported to have a sensitivity as low as 40% to 60% and, thus, cannot reliably be used to rule out an infection.[8-10] We might reasonably assume that each and every access attempt, no matter how brief or sterile in technique, introduces some risk of infection. Thus, in considering the balance of risk and benefit, we cannot recommend the routine and frequent sampling of CSF.[2,11,12] However, in some cases, sampling may be informative, such as when the clinical suspicion of infection is high, when response to antibiotic therapy requires monitoring, or when documentation is needed of no infection at the time of drain placement or removal.

When a decision has been made to access the EVD line, the following steps are taken. The rest of the CSF collection system is left open and draining. A neuroscience nurse is available during the access. Equipment needed for access is gathered, including sterile syringes of preservative-free sterile normal saline (usually two or three 10-mL syringes), three or four sterile red caps, two chlorhexidine swab sticks, medication to be administered in a prefilled syringe, two or three empty sterile 10-mL syringes, sterile gloves, a half drape, and a gown. The most proximal port is accessed in all situations.

First, don a face mask and hat. Then open all the equipment in a sterile fashion and lay it on the opened half drape. Save the plastic wrapper of the sterile gloves for later use. Using nonsterile gloves, hold the EVD line in the air with one hand and use a chlorhexidine swab stick to wipe the proximal access port, stopcock, and a fair length of EVD line proximal and distal to the port (Fig. 5.5A). Hold the EVD line aloft until it is completely air-dried, then place it on the inside of the plastic wrapping of the sterile gloves, which is also sterile. If you do not feel comfortable using the plastic wrapping of the gloves, you can use a second sterile half drape instead.

Don sterile gloves and a gown. Remove and discard the cap of the access hub (Fig. 5.5B). Use a second chlorhexidine swab to clean the inside of the port, the stopcock, and the EVD line a short distance proximal and distal to the port. Allow these items to dry. Attach the first empty syringe to the port, and turn the stopcock so that the port is open to the proximal EVD catheter. Clear the line of CSF from the port to the catheter tip by slowly drawing 1 mL CSF and setting it aside.

If the purpose of accessing the EVD is to draw cultures, attach two sterile 10-mL syringes and draw 3 mL of CSF in each. Because specialized studies may require more CSF, you should know the goal volume of CSF to be withdrawn before starting the procedure.

If the goal is to instill medication, attach the syringe with medications to the port after drawing and discarding 1 mL of waste (Fig. 5.5C). Slowly inject the medication. During the injection, keep an eye on the patient's vital signs. If concerns arise about vitals or if unexpected resistance is encountered, turn off the stopcock to the syringe and instruct the neuroscience nurse to turn the stopcock to the zero point on the CSF chamber to transduce ICP. If ICP becomes unexpectedly elevated, stop the injection, place a sterile red cap on the hub, perform a neurologic examination, and send the patient for an immediate computed tomogram (CT). When instilling thrombolytics, watch

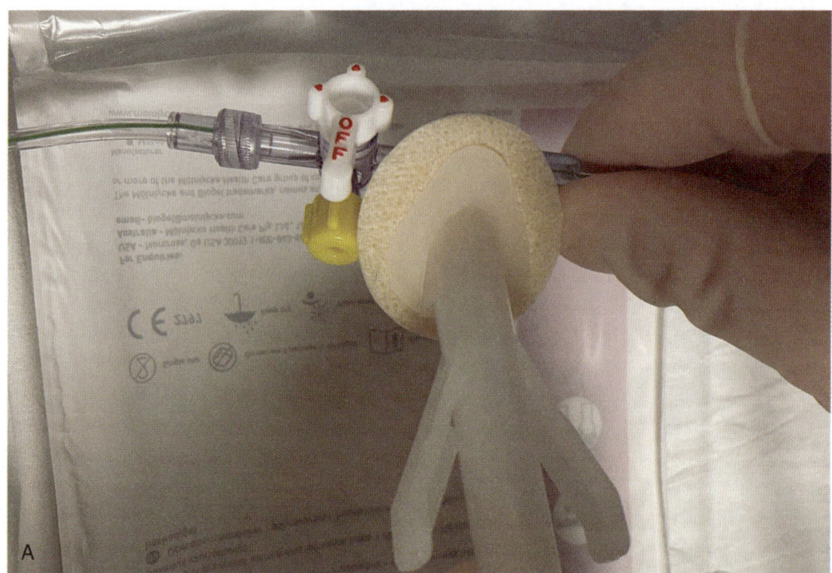

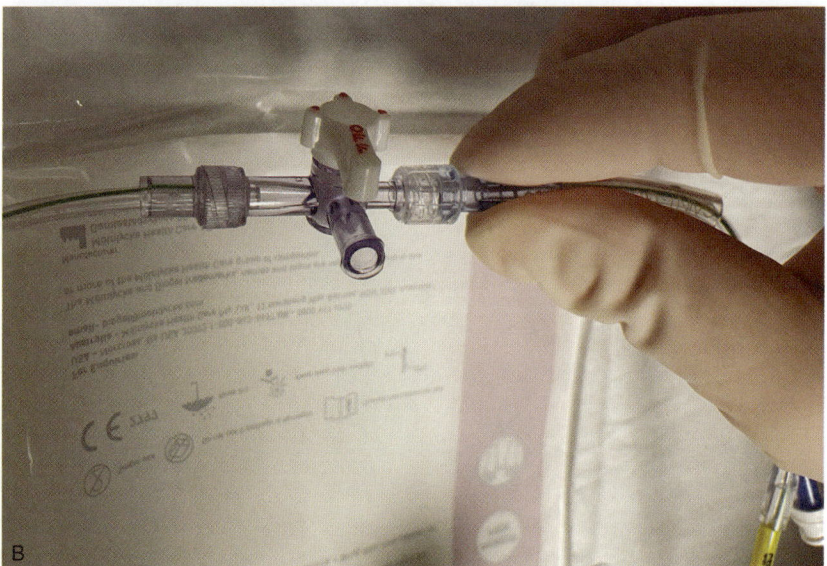

FIGURE 5.5. Steps to access an external ventricular drain (EVD) or a lumbar drain (LD) catheter. **A.** The proximal port of the EVD or LD is cleaned with sterile solution swabs. The inner surface of the sterile glove package is used as a stage. **B.** The port cap is removed and discarded. **C.** If medication is to be instilled or cerebrospinal fluid (CSF) drawn for cultures, a waste syringe is drawn, followed by use of the syringes containing medication and those to be sent for CSF cultures. **D.** The line is flushed distally to clear air bubbles. **E.** If necessary, a small amount of saline can be injected into the ventricles to clear debris. **F.** A new cap is placed.

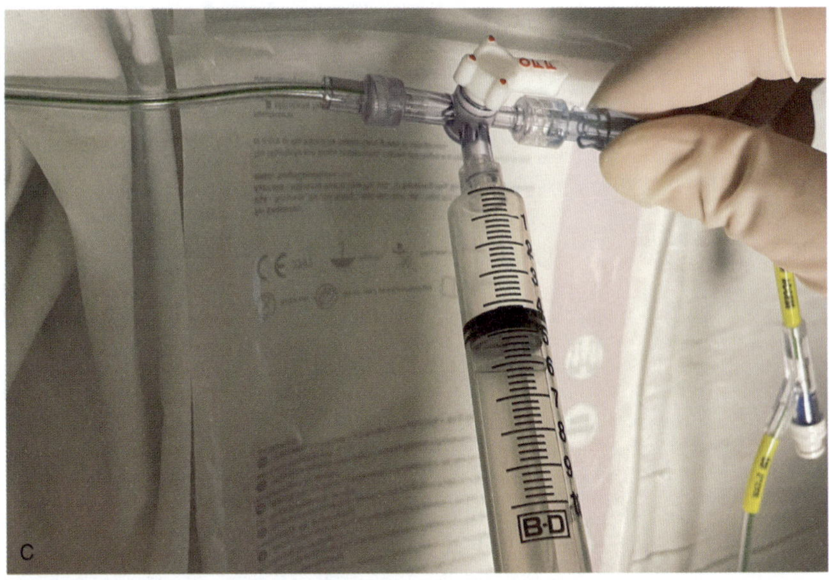

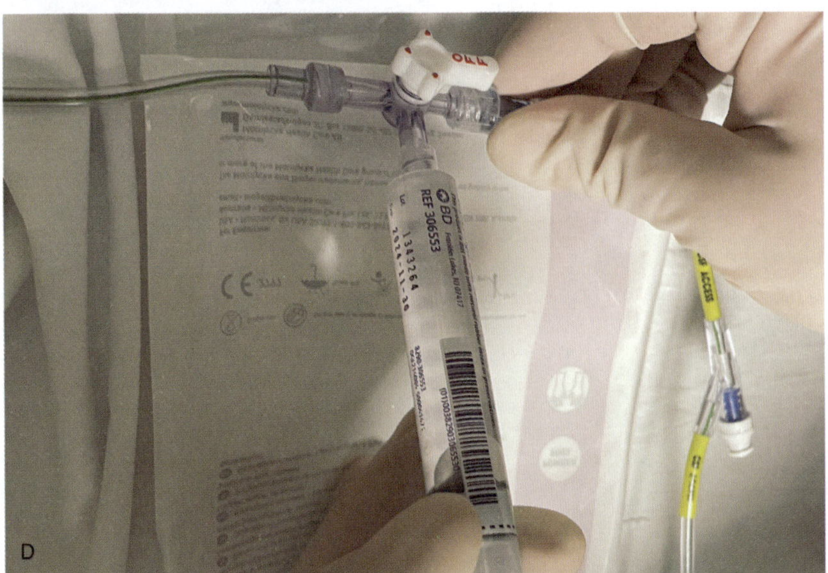

FIGURE 5.5. (Continued)

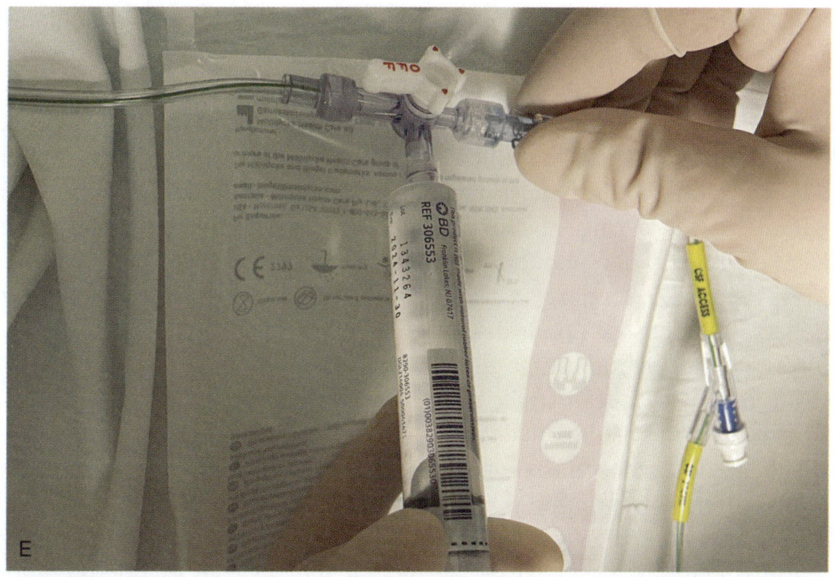

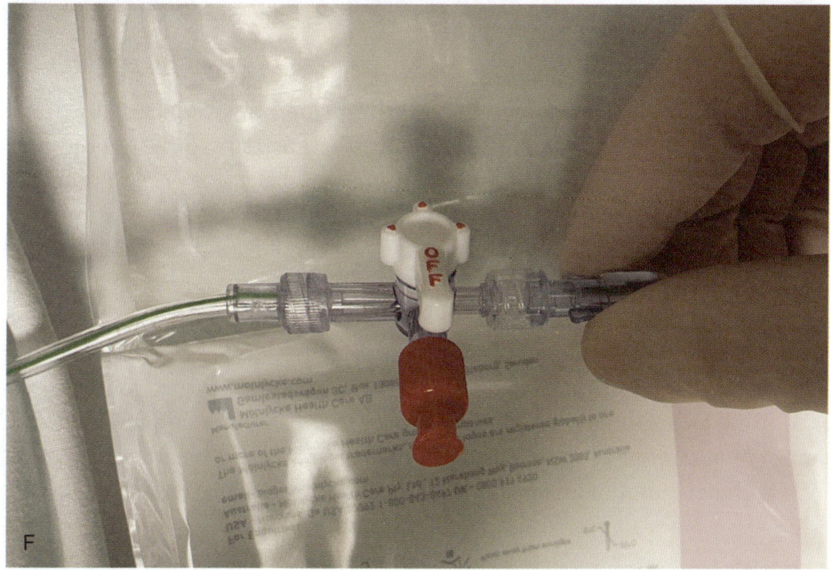

FIGURE 5.5. (Continued)

for suspected hemorrhage. When vasoactive substances such as nimodipine are injected too quickly, they can cause hypotension, requiring a pause during the injection. After the medication has been injected, inject 1 mL of sterile preservative-free normal saline to flush the medication into the ventricles. When medication must be instilled in a patient with borderline high or high ICP, the volume infused must match the volume withdrawn. Therefore, in that initial waste syringe, the total volume withdrawn should be equal to the volume of medication plus the 1 mL of saline needed to flush.

If the goal is to clear an obstruction, the location of the obstruction matters. If the obstruction is distal to the access hub, a waste syringe is not necessary. Rather, you can go directly to flushing distally into the Buretrol with a 10-mL syringe of sterile preservative-free normal saline (Fig. 5.5D). If the obstruction is proximal, you should first attach a waste syringe. You will likely encounter some resistance to withdrawing CSF. The degree of vacuum suction applied to the syringe should be based on your level of comfort and experience. Overaggressive vacuum suction can be dangerous, sucking brain tissue into the catheter or causing a hemorrhage. If suction does not bring air bubbles or occlusive debris into the syringe, try flushing proximally (Fig. 5.5E). We recommend flushing with minimal amounts of saline because overinjection can cause increased ICP, brain tissue dissection, and hemorrhage. You can also try flushing with thrombolytics in select patients when an unsecured vascular lesion, a recent hemorrhage, or a craniotomy is not a concern. Any resistance to injection should be a stopping point, and if new resistance develops with the elevation of ICP, maneuvers similar to those discussed previously should be used. If these actions do not clear the obstruction, the procedure should be stopped and a sterile red cap placed on the port (Fig. 5.5F). You then must decide whether the EVD should be permanently removed or replaced. We do not recommend leaving an occluded EVD in place for a prolonged period in hopes that the obstruction will clear or to use it as a simple pressure transducer because the accuracy of the ICP cannot be guaranteed. None of these maneuvers should be attempted if the EVD catheter is not in an appropriate position on postplacement imaging.

EVD Catheter Exchanges

In patients who require an EVD but have an obstruction that cannot be cleared or an infection that is directly attributed to the drain, the treatment team may opt to replace the EVD catheter or to place an LD in cases of nonobstructive hydrocephalus. Although the burr hole and catheter tract already exist, a catheter exchange carries the same risks as the original procedure. Antithrombotic medications have to be selected, and laboratory tests ordered.

The routine exchange of catheters as a prophylactic measure has been debated. Wong et al[13] conducted a prospective randomized trial of routine catheter exchanges in EVD patients without CSF infection and found no difference in the rate of subsequent infection (4 of 51 [7.8%] patients with an exchange vs 2 of 52 [3.8%] patients without an exchange; $p = 0.44$) or any changes in outcome. Given the risk inherent in catheter exchanges and the low likelihood of subsequent improvement, we recommend against the routine exchange of catheters to prevent infection, in conformance with recommendations of the Neurocritical Care Society.[2]

To prepare for a catheter exchange that is deemed necessary, you should first study prior imaging and determine trajectory and depth. We recommend using a completely new EVD setup, as for an original placement. Open the old incision and place a retractor. Pass a trocar, with the tip protected, to a new skin exit site. Use smooth tooth forceps to hold the catheter in place at the bone exit site. Pull the distal part of the catheter through from the skin exit site to the incision. Place a red cap on the clear plastic hub on the end to prevent CSF loss. When the time comes to remove the occluded catheter and pass the new one, do so in quick succession to ensure that the tract stays open. Lightly pull on the old catheter; if it does not give, do not pull it forcefully, which may result in hemorrhage. Insert the metal stylet into the old catheter to sever debris attached to the inside of the catheter. Rotate the catheter slightly instead of pulling it. When the old catheter tip nears the entrance into the parenchyma, prepare the new catheter in your dominant hand with the stylet in place. Identify the existing parenchymal hole, and advance the new catheter with very little forward pressure. If you encounter more than a little resistance, the catheter may be creating a new tract. This new tract may enter into the ventricle regardless, or it may be misdirected as covered in Chap. 2 ("Anatomy"), which will require revision. Remove the stylet at 5 cm and advance the catheter. When the catheter is at the appropriate depth, check CSF flow. If there is no flow, perform troubleshooting as highlighted in Chap. 4 on the procedural steps of placing an EVD or LD. Use the trocar to pass the catheter. Irrigate and close the incision, then secure the catheter. As with an initial EVD placement, obtain a CT to double-check placement.

EVD Transport

An EVD is at high risk of disconnecting or dislodging during the transport of a patient (Figs. 5.6 and 5.7). Before every transport, the treatment team must decide on a plan for protecting the EVD. Typically, in a patient who has had stable and normal ICP, the EVD can be shut off without draining. For short transports, the transduction of ICP is also unlikely to be necessary. Depending on the patient's clinical condition, monitoring should be continued and escalated. If the patient has been neurologically stable without ICP elevation but transport will be long, such as from one facility to another, then ICP monitoring should be continued. If the patient has elevated ICP, the position of the patient during transport should be discussed. If the patient will be lying flat, a lay-flat trial should be performed prior to transport. This trial should extend for several minutes. For patients with elevated ICP, we recommend monitoring ICP with the head of the bed elevated and continued ability to drain CSF. Longer transports of patients with high ICP may also require planning for medication administration. Patients with uncontrollable ICP elevation despite medical therapy (ie, tier 3) should not be transported.

During transport, one person should always be available to monitor the EVD to ensure that it does not get caught or pulled (Fig. 5.6A). Before a patient is transferred from bed to bed, a cleared path for the EVD line

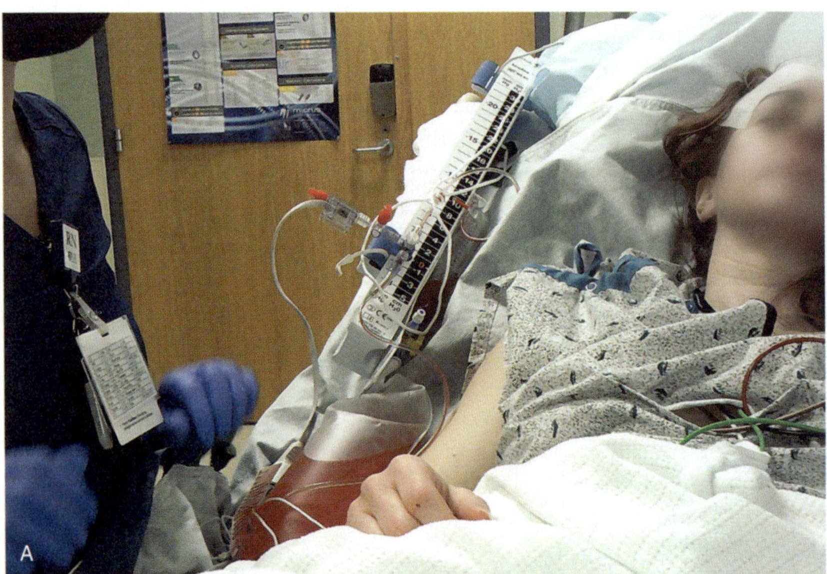

FIGURE 5.6. Patient transport or transfer. **A.** Both the external ventricular drain (EVD) and the lumbar drain (LD) are at risk of disconnection or dislodging during patient transport and patient transfers. A care team member is assigned the role of focusing solely on the EVD or LD collection system. During the pretransport or pretransfer checklist, the collection system is removed from the pole it is transferred with, clearly isolated, and cleared from entanglement with other lines and drains. **B.** The care team member assigned to the EVD or LD collection system maintains slack in the lines during transport or transfer, observes the lines to ensure that nothing is ensnared, and keeps the system upright. The EVD or LD collection system is then handed off to another team member or the dedicated team member walks it over to the pole where the system will be reconnected.

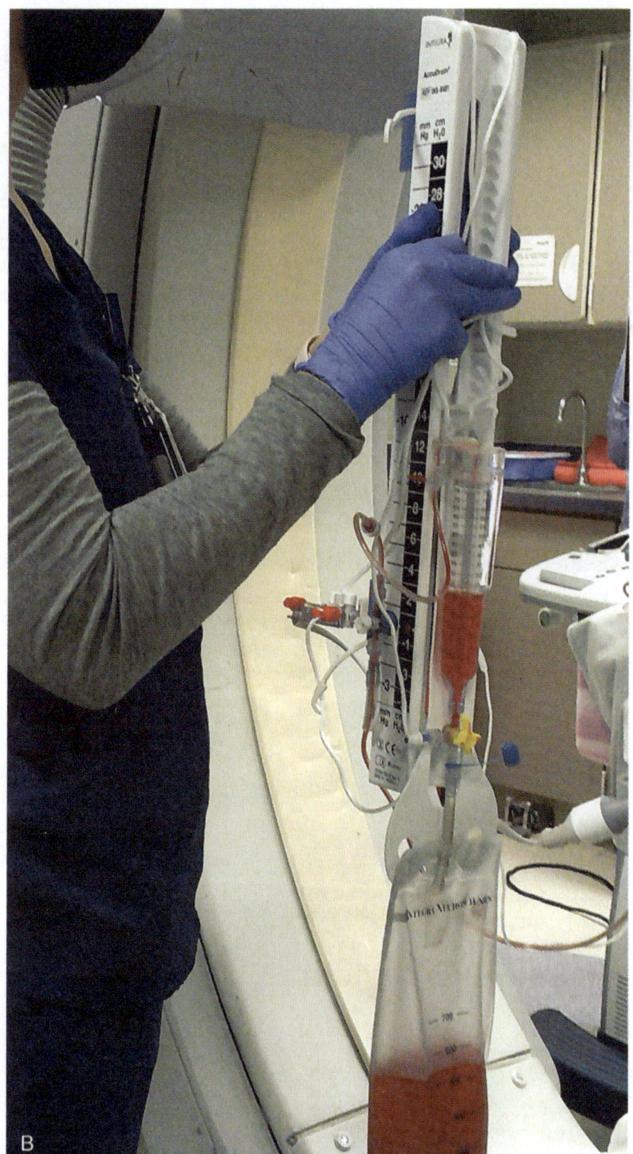

FIGURE 5.6. (Continued)

should be ensured, and the EVD line should have enough slack to accommodate the transfer (Fig. 5.6B). EVDs have been pulled out by lines getting caught on door handles, trapped between beds, and wrapped around other medical equipment or poles.

The potential air transport of patients with EVDs or LDs requires special consideration. The data are scarce, but one case report of a patient

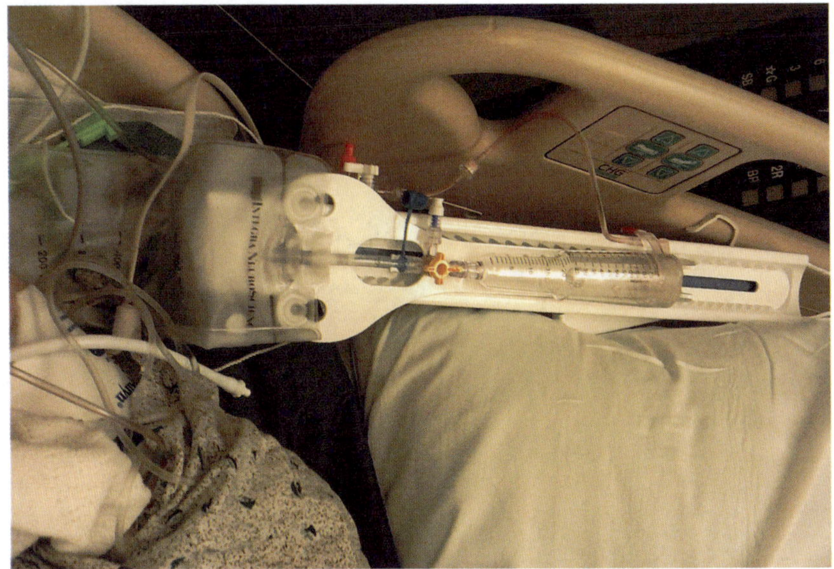

FIGURE 5.7. Inappropriate transport. This photograph illustrates an inappropriate way of transporting an external ventricular drain (EVD) or a lumbar drain (LD) collection system. Note that the pressure transducer is resting against the bedrails, where it can easily be fractured or bent. Multiple other lines are tangled with the collection chamber line. This setup can result in the inadvertent pullout of the EVD or LD catheter should traction be applied to the lines.

undergoing intracranial monitoring during flight documented a decrease in atmospheric pressure from 767 to 746 mm Hg that produced a concomitant increase of 10 mm Hg in ICP.[14] Thus, when air transport is necessary, we recommend continuous monitoring of ICP.

CSF Leak and EVD Pullout

When a CSF leak develops, your first task is to determine the location of the leak. In cases of a broken or faulty connecting hub, you should replace the entire system. If the damage occurs at the connection of the catheter to the CSF collection system, you can trim the catheter and place a new cap in a sterile fashion. If you discover a hole in the catheter where there is too little remaining tubing to trim, then you should replace the entire catheter. If you discover a leak from the catheter skin egress site, then you should place an additional purse-string stitch in a sterile fashion. This stitch must be deep and should gather a substantial amount of tissue. The goal of the stitch is to bring tissue snugly around the catheter. You must be exceptionally careful in placing this second stitch because the subgaleal route of the catheter may not be obvious, which can lead to the puncture of the catheter. If you find CSF at the site of the incision, the galeal layers were likely not well approximated at first closure or the catheter was punctured during closure. In such cases, you should then open the incision in a sterile fashion as if placing a catheter, explore it and the length of visible catheter, then replace the catheter if a problem is found or reclose the incision, ensuring that the galeal tissue is approximated on both sides.

Other causes of leakage should be investigated in patients who have a drain that leaks a second time after being oversewn for an initial leak. If a CSF leak occurs during the EVD weaning process while it is still clamped, the patient likely has hydrocephalus. You should unclamp the EVD and plan for conversion to a shunt. If the EVD has already been removed and CSF is leaking, you might consider multiple high-volume lumbar punctures with fenestration of the dura, an LD, or a transition directly to a shunt. If the second leak occurs while the EVD is in place and still draining, you should remove the EVD and place it in a different location or also place an LD.

If you can quickly identify a CSF leak, prophylactic antibiotic coverage is not required. However, when a leak is prolonged or its duration is unknown, it would be reasonable for you to order CSF cultures and add antibiotic coverage in the interim. Alternatively, you can send CSF cultures, but order antibiotics only if an organism is identified. The choice of antibiotics is institution-dependent but should focus on skin microbiota, gram-negative coverage, and fungal coverage.

If an EVD is inadvertently disconnected where the catheter joins the line, you can place a metal clamp on the catheter to halt CSF egress as distal as possible. The clamp is left in place, and the catheter is sterilized before it is attached to a new collection system. If you remove the entire EVD catheter, use a sterile gauze bandage to exert firm pressure on the exit site until appropriate closure can be performed.

EVD Weaning

The duration of the need for a drain and the weaning process are topics of debate. One prospective trial that used surveillance cultures determined that the duration of the drain was not a significant factor in patients who developed infections.[15] No prospective controlled trials exist, and definitive recommendations cannot be made on the basis of multiple retrospective studies with differing definitions of infection. Again, we follow the recommendations of the Neurocritical Care Society and suggest that the drain should be removed as soon as clinically possible; however, you should avoid preemptive removal necessitating lumbar punctures or a shunt.[2]

Once you have decided to remove the drain, the weaning process varies. A 2004 prospective randomized controlled trial compared fast (24 hours) and slow (>4 days) EVD weaning periods.[16] This trial found no difference in shunting between the two groups, but the slowly weaned group had a longer stay in the intensive care unit. We therefore recommend weaning as quickly as clinically possible. When deliberating whether to remove the drain, you can compare a head CT obtained prior to drain removal to previous imaging. This imaging can also serve as a baseline should hydrocephalus become a question after drain removal. As mentioned previously, you can also order CSF cultures at the time of drain removal.

Drain removal should be done in a sterile fashion after reviewing the patient's imaging and antithrombotic medication usage. When these medications are held and restarted is discussed further in Chap. 6, on complications. The necessary equipment includes a sterile half drape, chlorhexidine swab sticks, sterile gloves, sterile scissors, forceps, a needle driver, and sutures. Cut the sutures holding the EVD in place. Prep the egress site and allow it to air-dry. Gently tug on the catheter and pull with even pressure until the tip comes out. Check the tip to ensure that it is intact. Then use a dissolving monofilament suture to form a figure 8 stitch. Closure requires deep substantial bites of tissue and a strong knot. If the catheter will not move when tugged, despite reasonable pulling force, it may have been sutured in at the incision. To avoid the risk of tearing the catheter and leaving a retained part behind, you must open the incision and pull the proximal catheter out of the parenchyma. If necessary, you can cut the catheter in half, so that it comes out in two pieces: the proximal end from the incision and the distal end from the skin egress site. After the catheter has been removed, place a sterile gauze drain cover sponge and tape it, then monitor the patient closely for a CSF leak.

LD MAINTENANCE

As noted in the Overview for this chapter, most concepts for postplacement EVD care also apply to LDs. Below, we address only the differences in postplacement care for LDs compared with EVDs.

Dressing

Unlike the nonocclusive drain sponges we prefer for EVDs, large occlusive dressings are preferable for LDs (Fig. 5.8). An occlusive dressing for an LD is a must, given the relatively more difficult location to monitor and the proximity to potential contaminants. Despite the lack of strong

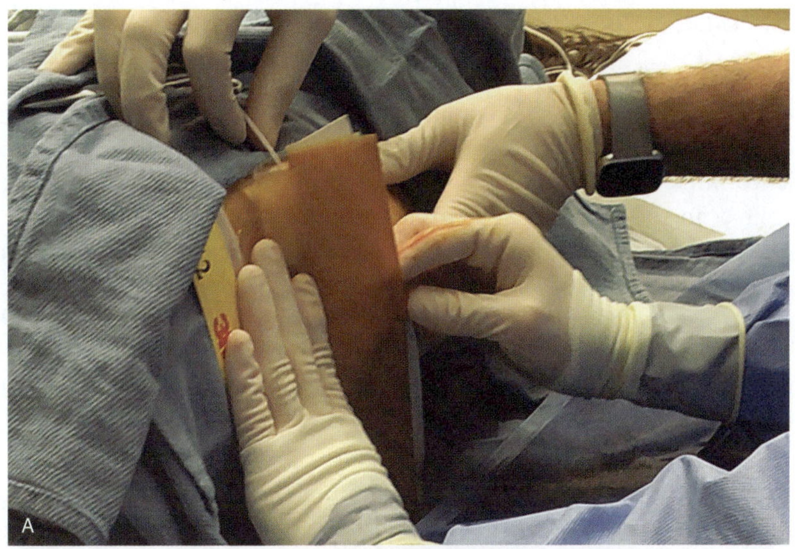

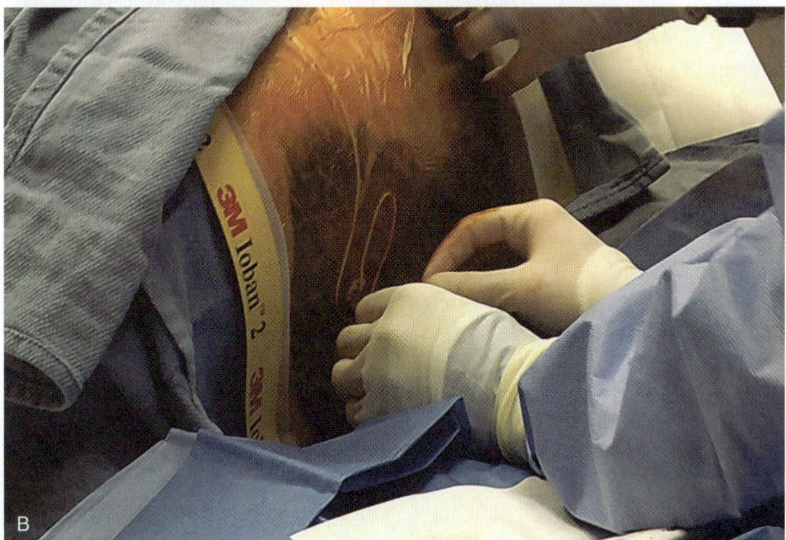

FIGURE 5.8. Lumbar drain (LD) dressing. We have transitioned to using Ioban as the occlusive dressing for patients with LDs. **A.** At placement and during dressing changes, sterile gloves are donned, and the site is cleaned with sterilizing solution. After the site has air-dried, the drain is held in a position to be free of kinks. **B.** Positioning the LD catheter appropriately allows for the even and accurate placement of the occlusive dressing.

data for Ioban (3M), we believe that it provides additional benefit over a plain occlusive dressing. This dressing should be changed infrequently unless it has lost its occlusive properties or becomes soiled. In contrast, the BioPatch is changed every 7 days.

CSF Collection Chamber and Positioning

For LDs, we use the same CSF collection chamber as for EVDs. Unlike drainage patterns for EVDs, we use only one type of drainage pattern for LDs. The drain is kept clamped at all times. Once every hour, the neuroscience nurse opens the drain and allows a prespecified amount of CSF to collect in the chamber. The drain is immediately closed afterward. If the drainage is slow, the collection chamber may be held low, close to the floor. We typically start at 10 mL every hour, regardless of the pathology. This process can be tailored to the ICP or the condition of the patient. The chamber is zeroed to the patient's tragus as is done for an EVD. The location of the Buretrol (ie, the draining pressure) is not important because the drain is always kept clamped.

Patients with LDs can be seated in any position. An elegant study in the subarachnoid hemorrhage population used benchtop experiments and computer flow simulations to show that the upright position maximizes drainage of the cranial compartment.[17] This investigation reinforces the fact that LDs can serve to optimize treatment options for patients with aneurysmal subarachnoid hemorrhage.

ICP, CPP, and Waveforms

Unlike an EVD, which typically drains continuously and forfeits real-time ICP monitoring, an LD will continuously read ICP because the default position is off and no CSF is draining. As long as there is no obstruction, the ICP recorded at the level of the tragus using an LD will be equivalent to the ICP recorded at the tragus with an EVD. An LD, unlike an EVD, will likely produce no waveform because of a combination of factors (Fig. 5.9). Unlike the spinal canal, the calvarium is nearly completely enclosed in bone, which dampens the pulsatile features of the waveform. Additionally, the waveform must transition from the large diameter chamber of the thecal sac to an LD tube with a much narrower diameter, then to a CSF chamber line with a larger diameter. Each of these transitions may dampen the waveform. However, with an accurate ICP, CPP will also be accurate.

CSF Sampling and LD Access

An LD is accessed for the same reasons and in the same manner as an EVD. Given the smaller diameter of the lumbar versus ventricular catheter, an LD will occlude more frequently than an EVD, especially in patients whose pathology, such as aneurysmal subarachnoid hemorrhage, produces substantial breakdown products in the CSF. However, clearing an obstruction

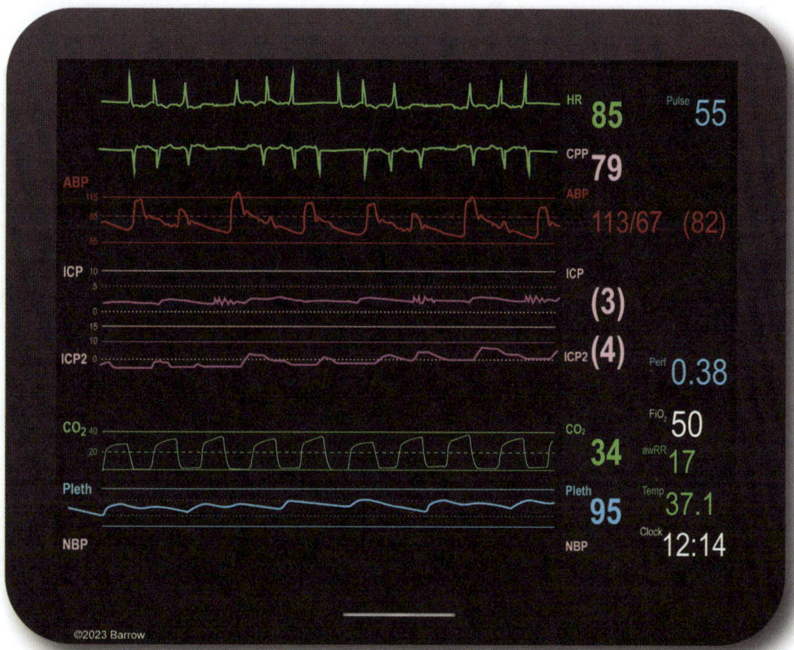

FIGURE 5.9. Concurrent external ventricular drain (EVD) and lumbar drain (LD) placement. This monitor shows readings from a patient who has both an EVD and an LD, with both leveled to the tragus. There is almost no intracranial pressure (ICP) waveform with the LD (ICP "(3)"), compared to that with the EVD (ICP2 "(4)"). However, the pressure readings are congruent. ABP, ambulatory blood pressure; awRR, airway respiratory rate; CO_2, carbon dioxide (capnography); CPP, cerebral perfusion pressure; FiO_2, fraction of inspired oxygen; HR, heart rate; NBP, noninvasive blood pressure; Perf, perfusion index; Pleth, plethysmograph waveform; Temp, temperature (°C).

in an LD or injecting medication proximally need not engender the same amount of trepidation as with an EVD. The spinal canal volume is much larger than that of the lateral ventricles, and there is little likelihood that the tip of the catheter will damage a nerve root or the conus medullaris with injection. With an open tip lumbar catheter, any debris that cannot be aspirated can be flushed directly into the lumbar cistern.

LD Catheter Exchanges

LD catheters should not be routinely replaced. Although obstruction from debris is more likely than with an EVD, the use of an open tip catheter in an LD will facilitate clearance of the obstruction more readily than with an EVD catheter. Thus, replacing the catheter is less likely and usually will be necessary only if the drain is the source of an infection or there is a break in the catheter at the site of its exit from the skin.

LD Transport

An LD is as much at risk of disconnection or dislodgement during patient transport as an EVD. Like patients with EVDs, patients with LDs should be evaluated for neurologic stability. The length of the transport should also dictate whether ICP should be monitored and CSF drained.

CSF Leak and LD Pullout

The more dependent the location of the entrance site, the more likely a CSF leak is, especially in patients sitting upright with the head of the bed elevated. This increased likelihood of a leak occurs because the fluid column of CSF experiences more pressure at the bottom of the spine than at the top. To determine the pressure of CSF at the drain exit site in the lumbar region with the head of the bed elevated, you can simply drop the zero point of the collection chamber so that it is level with the exit site. The resulting "ICP" will be the pressure in the thecal sac at the exit site. Luckily, the increased thickness of the tissue mass in the lower back helps to bolster against CSF leaks.

If you discover a leak with an LD that is still in use, you can attempt a second stitch. Place the suture in a sterile fashion, and cover it with a fresh occlusive dressing. As with an EVD, the goal of the stitch is to gather tissue snugly around the catheter but not to make it so snug that the tissue becomes necrotic. The amount of drainage per hour can also be increased.

If a leak occurs during the clamp and weaning trial, this is a sign, similar to that with an EVD, that the trial was not successful. You can attempt the placement of a second stitch. If the leak persists, you should initiate plans for a permanent shunt.

When a leak occurs after you have removed an LD, it may be a sign of hydrocephalus, as it would be in a patient with an EVD. In addition to ordering repeat intracranial imaging, you can make multiple high-volume lumbar punctures. Alternatively, you can replace the LD or you can place an EVD until a permanent shunt can be scheduled.

The same theory of antibiotic coverage applies for patients with LDs as for those with EVDs.

LD Weaning

As for patients with EVDs, those with LDs should be weaned as quickly as clinically possible. Given the current lack of antibiotic-coated lumbar catheters, and the more frequent access necessary to clear catheter obstructions, patients with LDs probably have an equivalent or a slightly higher risk of infection than patients with EVDs.[15]

ABBREVIATIONS

CPP, cerebral perfusion pressure

CSF, cerebrospinal fluid

CT, computed tomogram

EVD, external ventricular drain

ICP, intracranial pressure

LD, lumbar drain

MAP, mean arterial pressure

REFERENCES

1. Roethlisberger M, Moffa G, Fisch U, et al. Effectiveness of a chlorhexidine dressing on silver-coated external ventricular drain-associated colonization and infection: a prospective single-blinded randomized controlled clinical trial. *Clin Infect Dis.* 2018;67(12):1868-1877. doi:10.1093/cid/ciy393.

2. Fried HI, Nathan BR, Rowe AS, et al. The insertion and management of external ventricular drains: an evidence-based consensus statement. A statement for healthcare professionals from the Neurocritical Care Society. *Neurocrit Care.* 2016;24(1):61-81. doi:10.1007/s12028-015-0224-8.

3. Hawryluk GWJ, Aguilera S, Buki A, et al. A management algorithm for patients with intracranial pressure monitoring. The Seattle International Severe Traumatic Brain Injury Consensus Conference (SIBICC). *Intensive Care Med.* 2019;45(12):1783-1794. doi:10.1007/s00134-019-05805-9.

4. Carney N, Totten AM, O'Reilly C, et al. Guidelines for the management of severe traumatic brain injury, fourth edition. *Neurosurgery.* 2017;80(1):6-15. doi:10.1227/NEU.0000000000001432.

5. Hawryluk GWJ, Rubiano AM, Totten AM, et al. Guidelines for the management of severe traumatic brain injury: 2020 update of the decompressive craniectomy recommendations. *Neurosurgery.* 2020;87(3):427-434. doi:10.1093/neuros/nyaa278.

6. Heldt T, Zoerle T, Teichmann D, Stocchetti N. Intracranial pressure and intracranial elastance monitoring in neurocritical care. *Annu Rev Biomed Eng.* 2019;21:523-549. doi:10.1146/annurev-bioeng-060418-052257.

7. Kirkness CJ, Mitchell PH, Burr RL, March KS, Newell DW. Intracranial pressure waveform analysis: clinical and research implications. *J Neurosci Nurs.* 2000;32(5):271-277. doi:10.1097/01376517-200010000-00007.

8. Schade RP, Schinkel J, Roelandse FW, et al. Lack of value of routine analysis of cerebrospinal fluid for prediction and diagnosis of external drainage-related bacterial meningitis. *J Neurosurg.* 2006;104(1):101-108. doi:10.3171/jns.2006.104.1.101.

9. Tissot F, Prod'hom G, Manuel O, Greub G. Impact of round-the-clock CSF Gram stain on empirical therapy for suspected central nervous system infections. *Eur J Clin Microbiol Infect Dis.* 2015;34(9):1849-1857. doi:10.1007/s10096-015-2423-9.

10. Neuman MI, Tolford S, Harper MB. Test characteristics and interpretation of cerebrospinal fluid Gram stain in children. *Pediatr Infect Dis J.* 2008;27(4):309-313. doi:10.1097/INF.0b013e31815f53ba.

11. Jamjoom AAB, Joannides AJ, Poon MT, et al. Prospective, multicentre study of external ventricular drainage-related infections in the UK and Ireland. *J Neurol Neurosurg Psychiatry.* 2018;89(2):120-126. doi:10.1136/jnnp-2017-316415.

12. Angulo M, Springer L, Behbahani M, et al. Improving ventriculostomy management: risk and cost reduction through a multidisciplinary approach. *World Neurosurg.* 2019;122:e1259-e1265. doi:10.1016/j.wneu.2018.11.025.

13. Wong GK, Poon WS, Wai S, Yu LM, Lyon D, Lam JM. Failure of regular external ventricular drain exchange to reduce cerebrospinal fluid infection: result of a randomised controlled trial. *J Neurol Neurosurg Psychiatry.* 2002;73(6):759-761. doi:10.1136/jnnp.73.6.759.

14. Herbowski L. From paradigm to paradox: divergency between intracranial pressure and intracranial pulse pressure during atmospheric pressure fall. A case study. *J Neurosurg Sci.* 2022;66(2):103-111. doi:10.23736/S0390-5616.19.04737-4.

15. Scheithauer S, Burgel U, Ryang YM, et al. Prospective surveillance of drain associated meningitis/ventriculitis in a neurosurgery and neurological intensive care unit. *J Neurol Neurosurg Psychiatry.* 2009;80(12):1381-1385. doi:10.1136/jnnp.2008.165357.

16. Klopfenstein JD, Kim LJ, Feiz-Erfan I, et al. Comparison of rapid and gradual weaning from external ventricular drainage in patients with aneurysmal subarachnoid hemorrhage: a prospective randomized trial. *J Neurosurg.* 2004;100(2):225-229. doi:10.3171/jns.2004.100.2.0225.

17. Tangen K, Narasimhan NS, Sierzega K, Preden T, Alaraj A, Linninger AA. Clearance of subarachnoid hemorrhage from the cerebrospinal fluid in computational and in vitro models. *Ann Biomed Eng.* 2016;44(12):3478-3494. doi:10.1007/s10439-016-1681-8.

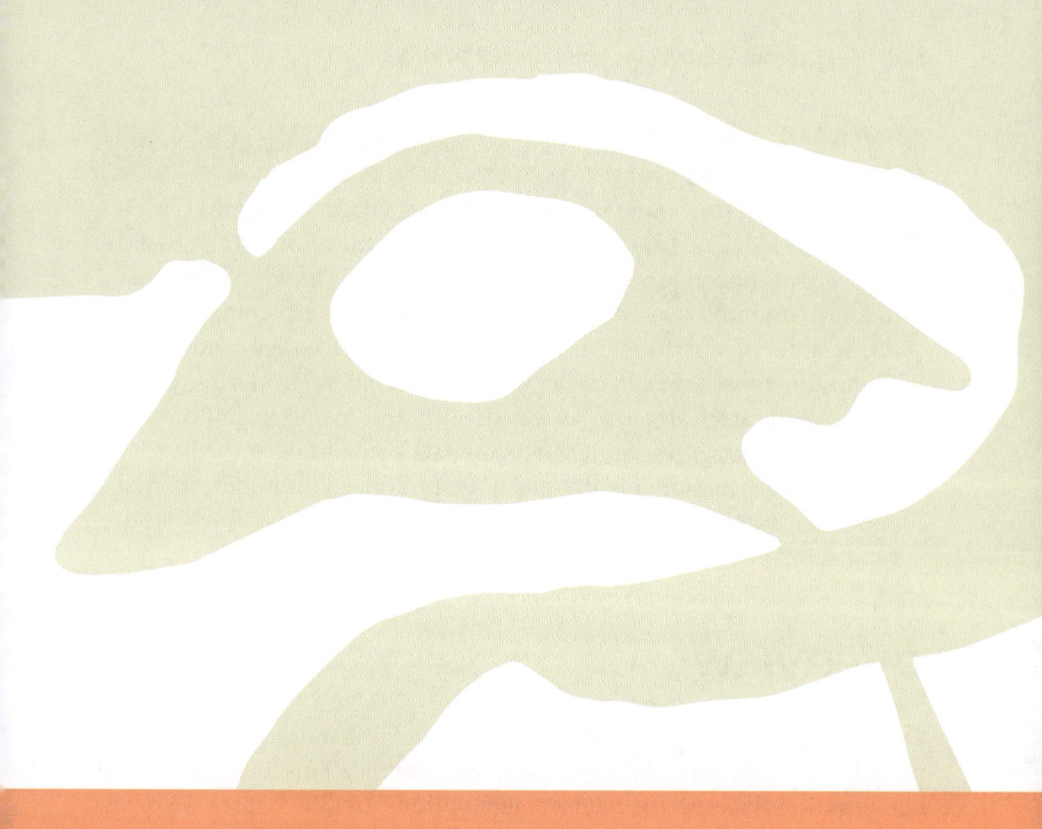

Complication Management

CHAPTER SUMMARY

Like any other procedure or device, external ventricular drain (EVD) and lumbar drain (LD) use can result in complications. You should be aware of the range of complications that can occur with both types of drains and follow existing protocols to manage each complication. Intracranial hemorrhage can occur with EVD placement, and spinal epidural hemorrhage can occur with LD placement. Both drains can also lead to infections such as ventriculitis and meningitis. If lumbar drainage is overaggressive, it can precipitate a subdural hemorrhage or even brain herniation. Finally, given the prolonged immobilization of patients with either an EVD or an LD or both, you must always keep venous thromboembolism in mind as an ever-present concern.

OVERVIEW

Once an external ventricular drain (EVD) or a lumbar drain (LD) has been placed, the care team must stay vigilant for complications. Each category of complications has specific management options. In this chapter, we review some of the more commonly encountered complications, how to prevent them, and how to deal with them when they do occur.

EVD COMPLICATION MANAGEMENT

Intracranial Hemorrhage

Intracranial hemorrhage (ICH) from EVD placement has been the topic of discussion largely in reports of observational studies. A baseline risk of approximately 1.1% for ICH has been reported for all craniotomies.[1] True hemorrhage rates associated with EVDs are difficult to calculate because of the differences in the types and timing of imaging after EVD placement. There is also the question of whether to define a hemorrhage as symptomatic or asymptomatic. Most of the reports in the neurosurgery literature group hemorrhages as tract or intraparenchymal, intraventricular, subdural, or some combination of these three types of hemorrhages (Figs. 6.1 and 6.2). The range of risk for all EVD-related hemorrhages is reported as 5% to 41%, whereas the range for symptomatic hemorrhage is ≤2.5%.[2–6] Of the symptomatic or larger hemorrhages, <1% typically require surgical intervention.[2,5]

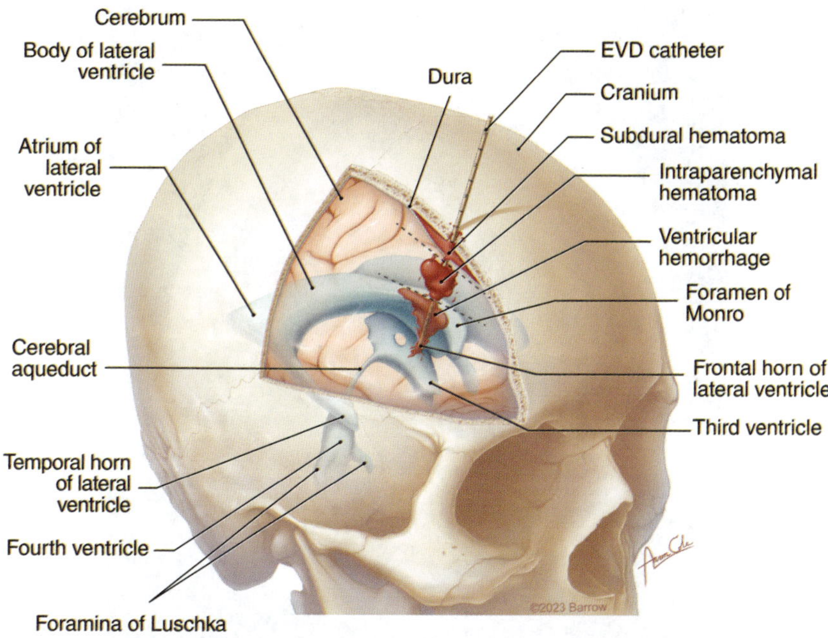

FIGURE 6.1. The typical locations of hemorrhage associated with external ventricular drain (EVD) placement are demonstrated, including subdural, intraparenchymal, and intraventricular.

If a new hemorrhage is identified on postplacement imaging, the typical next step is to repeat the imaging until the bleed is deemed stable. This evaluative process requires judgment gained with experience over time. A small tract hemorrhage usually can be noted without the need for further follow-up, whereas a patient with a large subdural hemorrhage with midline shift should be taken to the operating room without awaiting additional imaging. No standard interval has been established for repeat imaging, but it is typically 6 hours. When an intraventricular hemorrhage occurs, it may occlude the catheter. If imaging shows that the bleeding has stabilized, intraventricular tissue plasminogen activator can be considered.

Venous Thromboembolism

A major concern in any neurosurgery procedure, including a craniotomy, a spinal fusion, or placement of a cerebrospinal fluid (CSF) drain, is the timing to begin or restart antithrombotic medication. Neurosurgery patients are at increased risk of venous thromboembolism (VTE), either deep vein thrombosis (DVT) or pulmonary embolism, because of the immobilized or unresponsive state generated by many neurologic injuries. In one of the

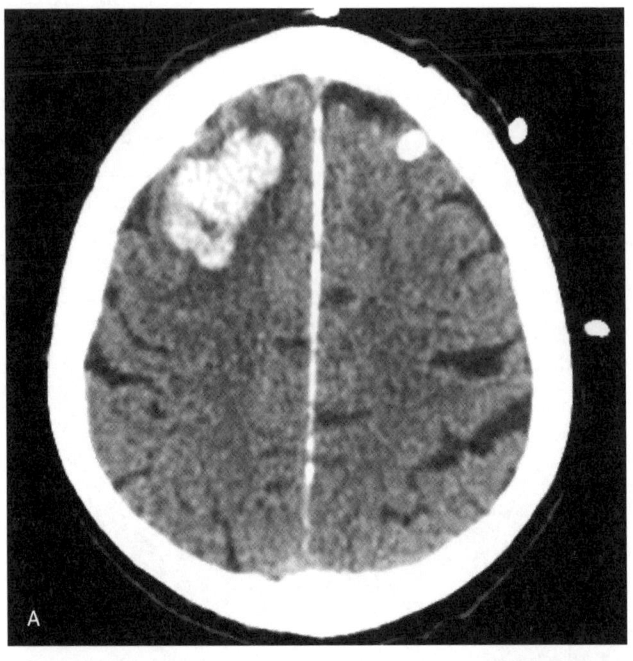

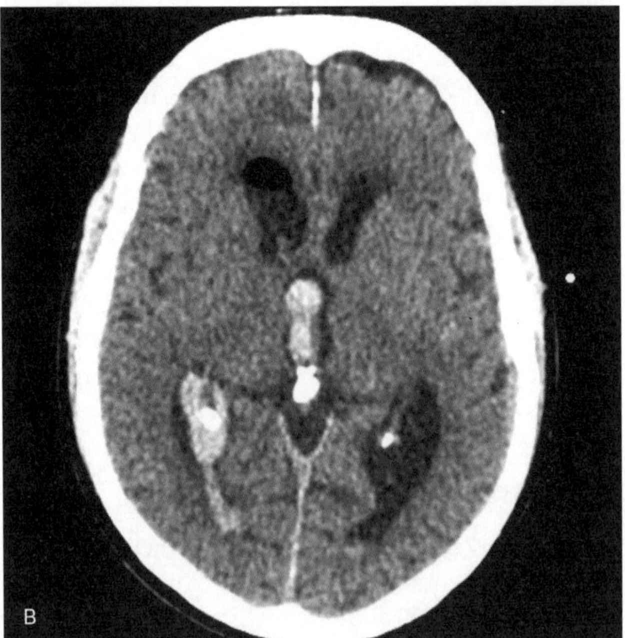

FIGURE 6.2. External ventricular drain (EVD) hemorrhage. Axial computed tomograms demonstrate a combination **(A)** intraparenchymal hematoma and **(B)** intraventricular hemorrhage after EVD removal. The patient underwent contralateral EVD placement and recovered.

most complete clinical practice guidelines, Gould et al,[1] on behalf of the American College of Chest Physicians, published an analysis in 2012 of VTE prevention in nonorthopedic surgery patients. They reported a 3.9% risk of clinically significant VTE at 30 days postcraniotomy for all indications. Patients with severe traumatic brain injury had a risk of up to 15%, those undergoing craniotomy for malignancy had a 7.5% risk, and those undergoing surgery for metastatic tumor had a 19% risk. In contrast, for patients with spinal surgery, the risk of symptomatic VTE at 91 days is 0.5% versus 2.0% for patients undergoing spinal surgery for malignancy. The baseline risk of major bleeding during spine surgery is less than 0.5%.[1]

Many published meta-analyses reviewing all the methods of VTE mitigation have not included trials with neurosurgery patients. Nevertheless, we summarize their results here because the principal findings have some bearing on neurosurgery patients. Table 6.1 summarizes the findings of the American College of Chest Physicians on VTE prophylaxis, as reported by Gould et al (2012).[1]

Given the low risk associated with the use of elastic stockings (ES) and intermittent pneumatic compression (IPC), which both offer clinically significant benefit, one might question whether the addition of pharmacologic prophylaxis is worthwhile. The relatively small number of randomized controlled trials and observational studies that included neurosurgery patients was analyzed in 2018 by Khan et al.[7] They found that pharmacologic prophylaxis produced an absolute risk reduction of 9% compared to placebo, with no increase in major or minor intracranial bleeding. Notably, only four of the nine studies had ES as a cointervention, limiting the usefulness of these findings. In a specific assessment of EVDs, Bruder et al[8] found an increased risk of ventriculostomy-related hemorrhage with the addition of anticoagulants or antithrombotics. It is important to note that the population in this retrospective study had prophylactic dosing with at least low-molecular-weight heparin (LMWH), and the authors were also assessing the effects of additional antithrombotic agents. Another group found no increased risk of hemorrhage with prophylactic anticoagulation.[9]

Therefore, our recommendation for patients with an EVD placement is to use at least IPC for prevention of VTE. For patients with a particularly high risk of VTE (ie, severe traumatic brain injury or malignant intracranial disease), the addition of pharmacologic prophylaxis should be considered, despite the minimal data on its risks and benefits. Whether low-dose unfractionated heparin (LDUFH) or LMWH is chosen is also contested between major professional society guidelines.[1,10] At the University of Rochester, we typically use LDUFH. Because VTE can take days to manifest, it is reasonable to wait for a short period before adding pharmacologic

TABLE 6.1: RECOMMENDATIONS FOR VENOUS THROMBOEMBOLISM PROPHYLAXIS FROM THE AMERICAN COLLEGE OF CHEST PHYSICIANS

VTE Prevention Comparison	Findings
ES vs no prophylaxis	ES reduce the odds of DVT by 65%
IPC vs no prophylaxis	IPC reduces the odds of DVT by 60%
LDUFH vs no prophylaxis	10,000-15,000 U/d of LDUFH reduces the odds of death from any cause by 18%, fatal PE by 47%, and nonfatal PE by 41%, and it causes a 57% increase in the odds of nonfatal major bleeding
LMWH vs no prophylaxis	LMWH reduces the odds of clinical VTE and PE by about 70% but doubles the risk of major bleeding
LMWH vs mechanical prophylaxis	LMWH reduces the risk of DVT by 80% and increases the risk of major bleeding by 57%
LMWH vs LDUFH	No difference in clinical VTE, PE, death from any cause, or major bleeding
Extended vs short-acting LMWH	Extended LMWH reduces the risk of all DVT by at least 50%
Fondaparinux vs LMWH	No difference in VTE, PE, or major bleeding
Fondaparinux with IPC vs IPC alone	Fondaparinux reduces any VTE by 69% but major bleeding is considerably more likely
Aspirin vs no prophylaxis	Aspirin reduces nonfatal DVT by 28% and fatal PE by 58%
Mechanical and pharmacologic prophylaxis vs pharmacologic prophylaxis only	ES with additional pharmacologic prophylaxis reduces risk of DVT by at least 60%
IVC filter vs no IVC filter	IVC filter reduces the odds of PE by 78% but has an 87% increase in DVT by 2 years

DVT, deep vein thrombosis; ES, elastic stockings; IPC, intermittent pneumatic compression; IVC, inferior vena cava; LDUFH, low-dose unfractionated heparin; LMWH, low-molecular-weight heparin; PE, pulmonary embolism; VTE, venous thromboembolism.

Data from Gould et al, 2012.[1]

prophylaxis to IPC.[11,12] We typically wait 24 hours after an EVD or a craniotomy with an EVD but modify this time frame depending on the clinical circumstances. When a patient has presented with ICH from a vascular lesion, securing or resecting the vascular lesion may be necessary before pharmacologic prophylaxis can be added. One study found no association between the type of preoperative ICH, the type of pharmacologic agent used for postoperative prophylaxis, or the rehemorrhage rate.[13] Whether to add postcraniotomy pharmacologic VTE prophylaxis and, if so, which type, would be an ideal topic for a large multicentered, multiarm, placebo, double-blind, controlled trial or for a large prospective observational analysis. Using more nuanced testing, such as thromboelastography to determine the risk of treatment and the response to it would also be a worthy addition to such a trial or observational study.

One last consideration is what to do in cases when a VTE develops after a craniotomy or an EVD placement. The typical treatment paradigms involve an unfractionated heparin (UFH) drip, LMWH, warfarin, or a novel oral anticoagulant (NOAC). In a 2017 meta-analysis of patients with cancer, Rojas-Hernandez et al[14] found that LMWH therapeutic anticoagulation did not increase the risk of ICH compared to warfarin. Important exclusion criteria of studies were craniotomy within 7 days or a known cranial vascular malformation. Another meta-analysis of patients with central nervous system tumors found that anticoagulation with LMWH or warfarin did not increase the risk of ICH except in glioma patients.[15] It is unknown whether studies were included or excluded based on craniotomy. In a retrospective study, de Melo et al[16] assessed 53 patients in whom VTE developed after craniotomy for tumors, aneurysms, abscesses, and shunts; all 53 were receiving anticoagulants. The reported overall ICH rate of 7.4% (4/54) is much higher than the 1.1% discussed previously, but the timing to initiation of therapeutic coagulation did not affect this rate. Warfarin was associated with a 13% rate of ICH compared to NOACs with a 0% ICH rate ($p = 0.13$). In another review of 42 craniotomy patients with VTE, there was no measurable hemorrhage rate when therapeutic LMWH or a UFH drip was used as soon as the second postoperative day.[17] One group that reported their process of surveillance computed tomograms (CTs) for patients on a UFH drip found only 3 hemorrhages in 83 patients.[18]

At the University of Rochester, our typical protocol is to begin with a head CT when a VTE is found or at least 24 hours have passed since neurosurgery or EVD placement. If no hemorrhage is evident on the CT, we initiate a neurosurgery protocol heparin drip that involves no UFH bolus and targets a partial thromboplastin time of 60 to 80 seconds. After the partial thromboplastin time has been in this range for 24 hours, we obtain a second head CT. If this second CT also demonstrates no hemorrhage, we then transition the patient to longer-term therapeutic anticoagulation. Whether the anticoagulation is LMWH, an NOAC, or warfarin depends on the preferences of the patient and caregiver. If warfarin is selected, we continue the UFH drip until the international normalized ratio goal is reached. If the first head CT shows a hemorrhage, the start of the UFH drip is delayed based on the physical size and stability of the patient and repeat imaging. If the second head CT after initiation of therapeutic heparin shows a hemorrhage, the drip is discontinued until the hemorrhage is stable on repeat imaging. If a large hemorrhage occurs, the heparin is reversed. In patients with a life-threatening or saddle pulmonary embolism who are hypotensive or teetering on the verge of cardiopulmonary collapse, heparin reversal takes precedence, and these patients may benefit from pulmonary mechanical thrombectomy rather than slower therapeutic anticoagulation.

Intracranial Infection

The incidence of intracranial infection from ventriculostomy was discussed in Chap. 3 in our review of the steps in the procedure preparation process. These infections can be broadly categorized as consisting of meningitis, subdural empyema, abscess, or ventriculitis (Fig. 6.3). In addition to the

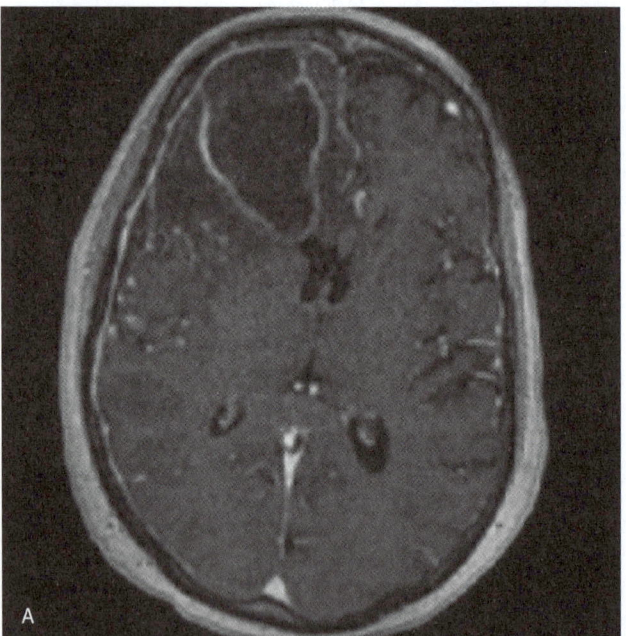

FIGURE 6.3. External ventricular drain (EVD) infection. **A.** Axial magnetic resonance imaging (MRI) demonstrates a contrast-enhancing intraparenchymal lesion in a patient who had an EVD placed during a previous admission and was readmitted with altered mental status. **B.** The intraparenchymal lesion appears bright on the diffusion-weighted axial MRI, which suggests infection. **C.** The fluid-attenuated inversion recovery axial MRI signal indicates significant swelling and mass effect. The patient underwent craniotomy and washout and recovered well.

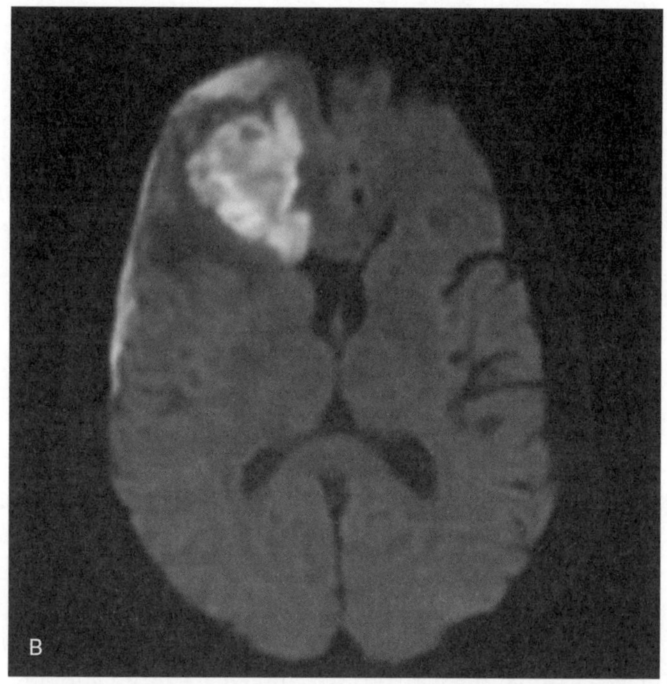

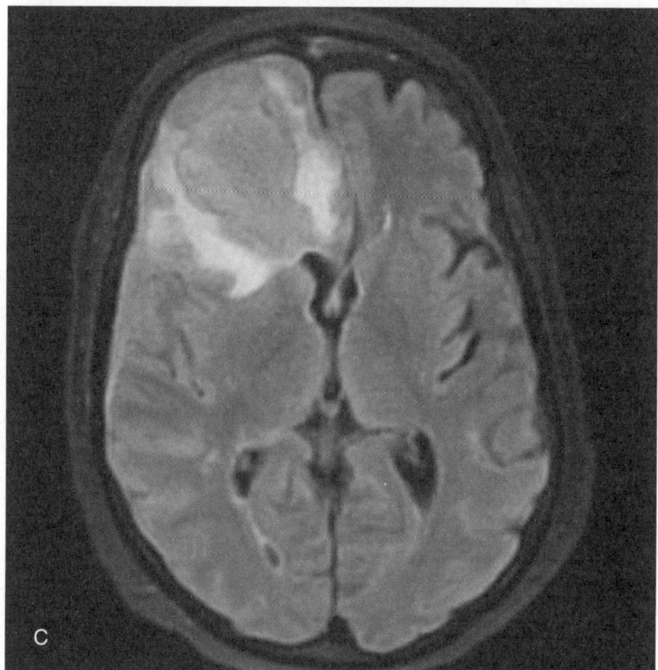

FIGURE 6.3. (Continued)

infection-control procedures performed at the time of drain placement, some treatment centers have implemented perioperative care bundles with the aim of reducing infection. Many aspects of these care bundles have been covered separately in previous chapters, reflecting the holistic approach required for both drains. A common aspect of many care bundles is a protocol or checklist.[19–21] Although a protocol or checklist can help reduce the likelihood of intracranial infection, adherence to either guideline over time is likely to decrease. Thus, both protocols and checklists require periodical reinforcement. Care bundles also contain instructions on hair removal, skin preparation, aseptic technique, catheter type, dressing factors, and the frequency of CSF sampling.[19–22] Perhaps the most telling study of care bundles was presented in a 2010 report by Harrop et al.[23] They presented a five-stage investigation of ventriculostomy-related infections (VRIs). Stage 1 was before implementation of any bundle. Stage 2 involved a protocol that called for elimination of traffic during the procedure, electric clipping of hair, skin disinfection, full sterile barrier protection, sterile placement technique, bio-occlusive dressing, and reduced CSF access. Stage 3 involved the same protocol but switched to an antibiotic-coated catheter. Stage 4 involved switching back to nonantibiotic-coated catheter while maintaining the protocol. The final stage involved reimplementing an antibiotic-coated catheter. The rates of VRI in each stage were 6.7%, 8.2%, 1.0%, 7.6%, and 0.9%, respectively. In an almost perfect adherence to the scientific method of removing and replacing the causative variable for effect, this study showed that an antibiotic-coated catheter is a key part of reducing VRIs.

Defining VRI is a matter of debate. A 2019 high-quality systematic review and meta-analysis by Dorresteijn et al[24] sheds reasonable light on some of the main considerations. In a review of 42 articles with 3035 patients, they found a ventriculitis rate of 23%. Fever was present in 72% of the patients with ventriculitis and in 29% without it. Headache was present in 62% and meningismus in 27%. A decline in consciousness occurred in 38% of the patients with ventriculitis and in 41% of those without it. CSF leukocyte count, CSF cell count, and CSF polymorphonuclear ratio cells were all inconsistently elevated in patients with ventriculitis. A mean protein concentration of 2.0 g/L was found in patients with ventriculitis versus 0.7 g/L in those without ventriculitis, with an area under the curve of 0.77 g/L when 0.8 g/L was used as the cutoff. The mean CSF glucose concentration was 52 mg/dL in patients with ventriculitis versus 100 mg/dL in those without ventriculitis. CSF lactate was inconsistently elevated, with an area under the curve of 0.90 mmol/L at a cutoff of >0.6 mmol/L. Dorresteijn et al[24] reported that we do not have enough data on CSF cytokines, except IL-6, to enable conclusions to be drawn. The mean blood leukocyte count in patients with ventriculitis was 17.8×10^9/L versus 12.2×10^9/L in those without ventriculitis. The mean C-reactive protein was 86 mg/dL in those with ventriculitis versus 48 mg/dL in those without ventriculitis, with a sensitivity of 100% at a cutoff of 22 mg/dL. These investigators also found that the causative organism was gram-positive cocci in roughly 60% of the cases and gram-negative bacteria in 32%. CSF culture positivity was 80% in patients with ventriculitis, but 27% of patients without ventriculitis had positive drain tip cultures or contamination. Gram stain was positive in 54% of patients with VRI and had a specificity of 85% to 100%. Compared to CSF cultures, a polymerase chain reaction of 16S rRNA had a sensitivity of 80%, a specificity of 98%, and a positive predictive value of 94%.

In 2017, the Infectious Diseases Society of America released their clinical practice guidelines for Healthcare-Associated Ventriculitis and Meningitis.[25] Table 6.2 summarizes their recommendations for the management of patients with these infections.

TABLE 6.2: RECOMMENDATIONS FOR MANAGEMENT OF HEALTHCARE-ASSOCIATED VENTRICULITIS AND MENINGITIS FROM THE INFECTIOUS DISEASES SOCIETY OF AMERICA

Topic	Recommendation
Red flag symptoms	• New headache, nausea, lethargy, seizures, or change in mental status
CSF sampling	• CSF cultures must be drawn and negative cultures held for 10 days for *Propionibacterium acnes* • CSF and blood cultures should be drawn before initiating antibiotics • Negative gram stain does not rule out infection • Drain should be sampled when removed with suspicion of infection • Drain should not be sampled when removed without suspicion of infection • Single or multiple positive cultures with clinical symptoms and abnormalities in counts indicate infection • Growth of an organism considered a contaminant and an asymptomatic patient with a normal CSF profile does not indicate a CSF infection
Specific CSF tests	• Detection of β–D-glucan and galactomannan may indicate fungal infection
Imaging	• MRI with gadolinium and DWI sequences is recommended for diagnosis

(Continued)

TABLE 6.2: RECOMMENDATIONS FOR MANAGEMENT OF HEALTHCARE-ASSOCIATED VENTRICULITIS AND MENINGITIS FROM THE INFECTIOUS DISEASES SOCIETY OF AMERICA (*Continued*)

Topic	Recommendation
Empiric antibiotics	• Vancomycin plus an antipseudomonal β-lactam antibiotic is recommended • Aztreonam or ciprofloxacin can be added for gram-negative coverage in patients with allergies to β-lactams • If a multidrug-resistant organism exists in the patient elsewhere, antibiotics should be modified accordingly
Narrowing antibiotics	• If MSSA, nafcillin or oxacillin can be given • If MRSA, vancomycin is used as first-line treatment or as alternative if vancomycin MIC is ≥1 μg/mL • In patients with β-lactam allergy, use linezolid, daptomycin, or trimethoprim–sulfamethoxazole • *P. acnes* can be treated with penicillin G • Gram-negative bacilli should be treated based on susceptibilities • *Pseudomonas aeruginosa* should be treated with cefepime, ceftazidime, or meropenem • *Acinetobactor* should be treated with meropenem, colistimethate, or polymyxin B if resistant • *Candida* can be treated with liposomal amphotericin B, often combined with 5-flucytosine • *Aspergillus* or *Exserohilum* can be treated with voriconazole
Intraventricular therapy	• Initiate when infection is poorly responsive to systemic antibiotics • Instill for 15-60 minutes, with dosage and interval based on CSF antimicrobial concentrations to 10-20 times the MIC of the causative organism
Duration of antibiotics	• Coagulase-negative *Staphylococcus* or *P. acnes* with mild symptoms: 10 days • Coagulase-negative *Staphylococcus* or *P. acnes* with systemic symptoms: 14 days • *Staphylococcus aureus* or gram-negative bacilli: 10-14 days • Continued positive cultures: 10-14 days after last positive culture
Catheter removal	• Remove and replace infected drain
Monitoring response	• Obtain CSF cultures, especially in patients with no clinical improvement

CSF, cerebrospinal fluid; DWI, diffusion-weighted imaging; MIC, minimum inhibitory concentration; MRI, magnetic resonance imaging; MRSA, methicillin-resistant *Staphylococcus aureus*; MSSA, methicillin-susceptible *S. aureus*.

Data from Tunkel et al, 2017.[25]

Limited high-quality prospective data exist regarding intraventricular and intrathecal administration of antibiotics; however, a few studies are noteworthy. Remeš et al[26] treated 34 postneurosurgery patients through either an EVD or an LD for meningitis or ventriculitis. The mean time to CSF sterilization was 2.9 days, with sterilization occurring slightly faster in the LD group (2.2 vs 2.6 days). The initial modified Rankin Scale score (mRS) was >2 in 94% of the patients, with 17 patients improving, 10 remaining the same, and 7 worsening or dying. Shofty et al[27] performed a propensity-matched historical analysis of data for 95 postneurosurgery patients who had carbapenem-resistant gram-negative bacteria. Systemic therapy with additional intrathecal or intraventricular therapy was administered to 37 patients, with the rest receiving systemic antibiotics only. After propensity matching, data were compared for 23 and 27 patients, respectively. Mortality was significantly lower in the intrathecal or intraventricular group (2/23, 8.7% vs 9/27, 33.3%) (odds ratio 0.19, 95% confidence interval 0.04-0.99).

LD COMPLICATION MANAGEMENT

Subdural Hematoma and Herniation

The most feared complication of LD is overdrainage leading to subdural hematoma and herniation. The incidence of ICH from LD use reported in the cardiothoracic and vascular literature is ≤3.5%.[28-31]

Motoyama et al[32] used propensity score matching to analyze two groups of 239 patients undergoing craniotomy. One group in the cohort underwent LD, whereas the other did not. The primary outcomes were brain herniation at 2 weeks and 30-day mRS scores. Brain herniation occurred significantly more often in the LD group (24/239 [10%] vs 8/239 [3%]; $p = 0.005$). Paradoxically, the LD group had outcomes superior to that in the group without LD. Outcomes were worse for patients in the LD group with brain herniation than for patients in the LD group without herniation. The authors determined that in both groups, the patients who had undergone decompression for a mass lesion from overdrainage fared worse.

In a 2021 publication, Lane et al[33] reported results for a single-surgeon operative series of 365 neurosurgery patients who also underwent lumbar punctures or placement of LDs. Not a single case of herniation was identified. In contrast, Wang et al[34] reported on a small series of eight patients with LDs who experienced herniation from overdrainage. These patients had a precipitous decrease in their Glasgow Coma Scale scores, with the time of onset of neurologic decline directly related to the speed of drainage.

Rapid recognition and corrective action brought about complete reversal of the condition within 24 to 48 hours in seven of the eight patients.

These results highlight the need for vigilance in managing patients with lumbar drainage. The subdural collection of CSF and brain herniation are rare events resulting from overdrainage that can be prevented with proper monitoring. In fact, because controlled lumbar drainage has been shown to be safe in patients with refractory intracranial hypertension,[35] it should be equally safe in other patients. We recommend always starting with a lower drainage rate. We typically prefer no more than 5 to 10 mL/hour. Intracranial pressure (ICP) transduction from the level of the tragus can help guide further therapy. If the patient tolerates this degree of drainage well but requires increased CSF drainage, the quantity per hour can be increased. Neuroscience nursing staff members should attend closely to the amount of drainage. The safest policy is to leave the drain clamped at all times unless it is being visually monitored for drainage. Although the LimiTorr (Integra LifeSciences Corp.) drain was recalled in 2019, similar concepts for limiting drainage would be worthwhile product advancements.

In the event that overdrainage occurs, the reaction must be swift. The drain should be clamped immediately. The head of the bed should be brought flat or placed in a reverse Trendelenburg position. If the patient develops cardiopulmonary instability or it continues, the patient should be resuscitated with appropriate measures, including endotracheal intubation, volume loading, atropine, and cardiopulmonary resuscitation. In such cases, a sterile technique should be used to access the LD catheter and up to 10 mL of preservative-free normal saline should be slowly injected. Once the patient is stable, imaging should be obtained. A large subdural mass presents a difficult situation. Numerous reports document paradoxical brain herniation with decompressive craniectomy.[36–38] The mechanism behind herniation is believed to be an already low-pressure intracranial system that is then subjected to atmospheric pressure after craniectomy. This pressure exerts downward force on the entire cranial structure, precipitating further herniation. If the patient has developed a large lesion that requires decompression, every attempt should be made to replace the bone flap at the end of the procedure.

Spinal Epidural Hematoma and Pharmacologic Prophylaxis

Spinal epidural hematoma (SEH) and pharmacologic prophylaxis can be considered in the same context. The incidence of SEH after LD placement has been documented in studies of thoracic and abdominal aortic repair, with a reported incidence of ≤3.2%.[28–31] In the obstetrics literature, the rate of SEH in patients undergoing neuraxial anesthesia is reported as 1:200,000 to 1:250,000.[39] In the anesthesia literature, SEH is reported to occur in <1:150,000 epidural cases and in <1:220,000 spinal anesthetic cases.[40]

The next question that arises is the effect of thromboprophylaxis or antithrombotic medications on the risk of SEH. The most extensive review on the topic comes from the 2018 evidence-based guidelines of the American Society of Regional Anesthesia and Pain Medicine (Table 6.3).[40]

TABLE 6.3: GUIDELINES FOR SPINAL ANESTHESIA IN PATIENTS ON ANTITHROMBOTIC MEDICATIONS FROM THE AMERICAN SOCIETY OF REGIONAL ANESTHESIA AND PAIN MEDICINE

Medication	Recommendation
Fibrinolytic/thrombolytic	• Wait 48 hours after last dose or until documented normalization of coagulation • If administered within 48 hours in emergency situations, perform neurologic checks at least every 2 hours
Unfractionated heparin infusion	• Discontinue heparin infusion 4-6 hours before needle placement or catheter removal • Delay heparin infusion for 1 hour after needle placement or catheter removal
Subcutaneous prophylaxis: unfractionated heparin	• Low dose (≤5000 U 3×/d): 4-6 hours after last dose for placement or removal of catheter • Medium dose (≤10,000 U 2×/d): 12 hours after last dose • High dose (>20,000 U): 24 hours after last dose
Low-molecular-weight heparin	• Prophylactic dosing: place catheter 12 hours after last dose; delay restarting for 12 hours after placement or 4 hours after catheter removal • Therapeutic dosing: place catheter 24 hours after last dose; delay restarting for 24 hours after placement or 4 hours after catheter removal
Anti-factor Xa	• Delay restarting for 6 hours after catheter removal
Direct Xa inhibitor	• Rivaroxaban: place catheter 72 hours after last dose; delay restarting for 6 hours after catheter removal • Apixaban: place catheter 72 hours after last dose; delay restarting for 6 hours after catheter removal • Edoxaban: place catheter 72 hours after last dose; delay restarting for 6 hours after catheter removal • Betrixaban: place catheter 72 hours after last dose; delay restarting for 5 hours after catheter removal

(Continued)

TABLE 6.3: GUIDELINES FOR SPINAL ANESTHESIA IN PATIENTS ON ANTITHROMBOTIC MEDICATIONS FROM THE AMERICAN SOCIETY OF REGIONAL ANESTHESIA AND PAIN MEDICINE (*Continued*)

Medication	Recommendation
Parenteral direct thrombin inhibitor	• Do not place catheter
Oral direct thrombin inhibitor	• Dabigatran: place catheter 72-120 hours after last dose (based on renal function); delay restarting for 6 hours after catheter removal
Vitamin K antagonist	• INR should be normalized before placement • INR should be <1.5 before catheter removal • With indwelling catheter while on medication, target INR <3.0 and watch closely
Antiplatelet agent	• NSAIDs: no need to withhold • Clopidogrel: place catheter 5-7 days after last dose; restart 24 hours after placement; restart immediately after catheter removal or 6 hours after loading dose • Ticlopidine: place catheter 10 days after last dose; restart 24 hours after placement; restart immediately after catheter removal or 6 hours after loading dose • Prasugrel: place catheter 7-10 days after last dose; restart 24 hours after placement; catheter should not be maintained while on therapy; restart immediately after catheter removal or 6 hours after loading dose • Ticagrelor: place catheter 5-7 days after last dose; restart 24 hours after placement; catheter should not be maintained while on therapy; restart immediately after catheter removal or 6 hours after loading dose • Glycoprotein IIb/IIIa inhibitor: abciximab 24-48 hours after last dose; eptifibatide or tirofiban 4-8 hours after last dose • Cilostazol: place catheter 48 hours after last dose; restart 6 hours after catheter removal • Dipyridamole: place catheter 24 hours after last dose; restart 6 hours after catheter removal • Cangrelor: place catheter 3 hours after last dose; restart 8 hours after catheter removal

INR, international normalized ratio; NSAIDs, nonsteroidal anti-inflammatory drugs.

Data from Horlocker et al, 2018.[40]

Although these anesthesia guidelines do not focus directly on LD, they are a more realistic comparator for EVD and LD patients than the spinal decompression or fusion guidelines.

In patients who undergo thoracic or abdominal aortic endovascular procedures, LDs are often placed prophylactically prior to heparinization. After the drain is in place, these patients undergo systemic heparinization with an activated clotting time goal of >250 seconds.[28] The low rate of SEH in this population, despite such heparinization, connotes the general safety of the drain despite the need for anticoagulation. However, the American Society of Regional Anesthesia and Pain Medicine guidelines include some interesting data documenting major increases in the incidence of SEH, depending on the timing of heparin administration.[40] In patients with epidural anesthesia, the incidence of SEH with heparinization in patients not previously receiving heparin increases from 1:220,000 to 1:70,000. The incidence is further increased to 1:8700 if an LD is placed within 1 hour of heparin administration. The importance of the LD placement technique is further highlighted because this incidence decreases even further to 1:2000 if there is a traumatic tap into the CSF space. One might argue that these data show that the technique conveys far more importance than anticoagulation in the prevention of SEH (relative risk 112 for traumatic vs 3.6 for atraumatic heparinized procedure).

A lumbar SEH typically occurs 2.6 days after an LD procedure, but the time frame can range from 0.8 to 5.0 days postprocedure.[41,42] Because of this variance in onset, the delayed presentation of new neurologic symptoms should be given serious consideration. Unlike patients with cervical and thoracic SEH, who are much more likely to present with complete paralysis (100% for each region), patients with symptomatic lumbar SEH have a rate of paralysis as low as 25%.[42] Conversely, patients with lumbar SEH are much more likely to present with acute and severe axial pain and radiculopathy, as well as bowel and bladder dysfunction.[41,42] The timing and symptoms are notable, especially in patients with LDs who have undergone thoracic or abdominal aortic repair. Patients with ischemic stroke to the spinal cord will present much more acutely with painless paralysis. If SEH is suspected, imaging should be obtained immediately.[41] Although an argument might be made that time can be saved by forgoing imaging, its benefits are twofold. First, imaging confirms the diagnosis made as a result of the clinical exam, and second, it also allows for operative planning of the size of the decompression.[41] SEH induced by an LD can be quite focal at the site of insertion or over many levels, which is not always apparent at surgery. Magnetic resonance imaging is the diagnostic modality of choice because it can readily discern the degree of neural compression and the extent of the hematoma.[41] Other imaging modalities such as computed tomography with contrast may have a higher false-negative rate, and computed tomography myelography is not emergently available in most institutions.[41] Once a diagnosis of SEH has been made, the primary management for patients with symptomatic SEH is surgical decompression and evacuation.[41] If the patient has only minimal pain or the SEH is incidental, conservative management can be considered. The timing of surgery has been a matter of debate, but good outcomes have been shown if surgery is performed within 6 hours of onset.[41] Approximately 50% of patients recover completely after SEH, with recovery influenced by such factors as timing to surgical decompression, preoperative neurologic function, and the speed at which deficits develop.[41]

Infection

The incidence of LD infection is reported to be 3% to 7% in retrospective data.[43–46] One prospective randomized trial identified an infection rate of 1.4%.[46] In patients with suspected meningitis, ventriculitis, or cerebritis, we follow the same recommendations that we do for EVD infections. We collect CSF and other cultures. We exchange the drain for either an LD at a different level or an EVD. If needed, we start the patient on intrathecal antibiotics.

Low–Intracranial Pressure Headaches and CSF Leak

Frank CSF leaks were covered in Chap. 5, which addresses troubleshooting. If a patient develops headaches consistent with low ICP, the initial investigation is a physical exam. Patients are often more comfortable when recumbent, and their headaches may begin shortly after they sit up or start to walk. A CSF leak may also be associated with neck pain, nausea, tinnitus, and emesis. Recumbency tends to quickly resolve these symptoms. We also examine the site of the LD and palpate it to ensure that there is no bogginess or fullness beneath the skin.

Typically, other diagnostic tests are not needed at this point. The patient may try caffeine to palliate symptoms, and a blood patch can be scheduled. If the first blood patch is not successful, a second and even a third should be scheduled. If symptoms still do not resolve, further investigation is necessary.

ABBREVIATIONS

CSF, cerebrospinal fluid

CT, computed tomogram

DVT, deep vein thrombosis

ES, elastic stockings

EVD, external ventricular drain

ICH, intracranial hemorrhage

ICP, intracranial pressure

IPC, intermittent pneumatic compression

LD, lumbar drain

LDUFH, low-dose unfractionated heparin

LMWH, low-molecular-weight heparin

mRS, modified Rankin Scale

NOAC, novel oral anticoagulant

SEH, spinal epidural hematoma

UFH, unfractionated heparin

VRI, ventriculostomy-related infection

VTE, venous thromboembolism

REFERENCES

1. Gould MK, Garcia DA, Wren SM, et al. Prevention of VTE in nonorthopedic surgical patients. *Antithrombotic Therapy and Prevention of Thrombosis, 9th ed: American College of Chest Physicians Evidence-Based Clinical Practice Guidelines. Chest.* 2012;141 (2 Suppl):e227S-e277S. doi:10.1378/chest.11-2297.

2. Kakarla UK, Kim LJ, Chang SW, Theodore N, Spetzler RF. Safety and accuracy of bedside external ventricular drain placement. *Neurosurgery.* 2008;63(1 Suppl 1):ONS162-166; discussion ONS166-167. doi:10.1227/01.neu.0000335031.23521.d0.

3. Ehtisham A, Taylor S, Bayless L, Klein MW, Janzen JM. Placement of external ventricular drains and intracranial pressure monitors by neurointensivists. *Neurocrit Care.* 2009;10(2):241-247. doi:10.1007/s12028-008-9097-4.

4. Maniker AH, Vaynman AY, Karimi RJ, Sabit AO, Holland B. Hemorrhagic complications of external ventricular drainage. *Neurosurgery.* 2006;59(4 Suppl 2):ONS419-424; discussion ONS424-425. doi:10.1227/01.NEU.0000222817.99752.E6.

5. Gardner PA, Engh J, Atteberry D, Moossy JJ. Hemorrhage rates after external ventricular drain placement. *J Neurosurg.* 2009;110(5):1021-1025. doi:10.3171/2008.9. JNS17661.

6. Dey M, Stadnik A, Riad F, et al. Bleeding and infection with external ventricular drainage: a systematic review in comparison with adjudicated adverse events in the ongoing Clot Lysis Evaluating Accelerated Resolution of Intraventricular Hemorrhage Phase III

(CLEAR-III IHV) trial. *Neurosurgery.* 2015;76(3):291-300; discussion 301. doi:10.1227/NEU.0000000000000624.

7. Khan NR, Patel PG, Sharpe JP, Lee SL, Sorenson J. Chemical venous thromboembolism prophylaxis in neurosurgical patients: an updated systematic review and meta-analysis. *J Neurosurg.* 2018;129(4):906-915. doi:10.3171/2017.2.JNS162040.

8. Bruder M, Schuss P, Konczalla J, et al. Ventriculostomy-related hemorrhage after treatment of acutely ruptured aneurysms: the influence of anticoagulation and antiplatelet treatment. *World Neurosurg.* 2015;84(6):1653-1659. doi:10.1016/j.wneu.2015.07.003.

9. Zachariah J, Snyder KA, Graffeo CS, et al. Risk of ventriculostomy-associated hemorrhage in patients with aneurysmal subarachnoid hemorrhage treated with anticoagulant thromboprophylaxis. *Neurocrit Care.* 2016;25(2):224-229. doi:10.1007/s12028-016-0262-x.

10. Anderson DR, Morgano GP, Bennett C, et al. American Society of Hematology 2019 guidelines for management of venous thromboembolism: prevention of venous thromboembolism in surgical hospitalized patients. *Blood Adv.* 2019;3(23):3898-3944. doi:10.1182/bloodadvances.2019000975.

11. Khaldi A, Helo N, Schneck MJ, Origitano TC. Venous thromboembolism: deep venous thrombosis and pulmonary embolism in a neurosurgical population. *J Neurosurg.* 2011;114(1):40-46. doi:10.3171/2010.8.JNS10332.

12. Tanweer O, Boah A, Huang PP. Risks for hemorrhagic complications after placement of external ventricular drains with early chemical prophylaxis against venous thromboembolisms. *J Neurosurg.* 2013;119(5):1309-1313. doi:10.3171/2013.7.JNS13313.

13. Farr S, Toor H, Patchana T, et al. Risks, benefits, and the optimal time to resume deep vein thrombosis prophylaxis in patients with intracranial hemorrhage. *Cureus.* 2019;11(10):e5827. doi:10.7759/cureus.5827.

14. Rojas-Hernandez CM, Oo TH, Garcia-Perdomo HA. Risk of intracranial hemorrhage associated with therapeutic anticoagulation for venous thromboembolism in cancer patients: a systematic review and meta-analysis. *J Thromb Thrombolysis.* 2017;43(2):233-240. doi:10.1007/s11239-016-1434-4.

15. Zwicker JI, Karp Leaf R, Carrier M. A meta-analysis of intracranial hemorrhage in patients with brain tumors receiving therapeutic anticoagulation. *J Thromb Haemost.* 2016;14(9):1736-1740. doi:10.1111/jth.13387.

16. de Melo Junior JO, Lodi Campos Melo MA, da Silva Lavradas LAJ, et al. Therapeutic anticoagulation for venous thromboembolism after recent brain surgery: evaluating the risk of intracranial hemorrhage. *Clin Neurol Neurosurg.* 2020;197:106202. doi:10.1016/j.clineuro.2020.106202.

17. Scheller C, Rachinger J, Strauss C, Alfieri A, Prell J, Koman G. Therapeutic anticoagulation after craniotomies: is the risk for secondary hemorrhage overestimated? *J Neurol Surg A Cent Eur Neurosurg.* 2014;75(1):2-6. doi:10.1055/s-0033-1345686.

18. Hacker E, Ozpinar A, Fernandes D, Agarwal N, Gross BA, Alan N. The utility of routine head CT for hemorrhage surveillance in post-craniotomy patients undergoing anticoagulation for venous thromboembolism. *J Clin Neurosci.* 2021;85:78-83. doi:10.1016/j.jocn.2020.12.010.

19. Kubilay Z, Amini S, Fauerbach LL, Archibald L, Friedman WA, Layon AJ. Decreasing ventricular infections through the use of a ventriculostomy placement bundle: experience at a single institution. *J Neurosurg.* 2013;118(3):514-520. doi:10.3171/2012.11.JNS121336.

20. Alunpipatthanachai B, Thirapattaraphan P, Fried H, Vavilala MS, Lele AV. External ventricular drain management practices in Thailand: results of the EPRACT Study. *World Neurosurg.* 2019;126:e743-e752. doi:10.1016/j.wneu.2019.02.144.

21. Baum GR, Hooten KG, Lockney DT, et al. External ventricular drain practice variations: results from a nationwide survey. *J Neurosurg.* 2017;127(5):1190-1197. doi:10.31 71/2016.9.JNS16367.

22. Camacho EF, Boszczowski I, Freire MP, et al. Impact of an educational intervention implanted in a neurological intensive care unit on rates of infection related to external ventricular drains. *PLoS One.* 2013;8(2):e50708. doi:10.1371/journal.pone.0050708.

23. Harrop JS, Sharan AD, Ratliff J, et al. Impact of a standardized protocol and antibiotic-impregnated catheters on ventriculostomy infection rates in cerebrovascular patients. *Neurosurgery.* 2010;67(1):187-191; discussion 191. doi:10.1227/01. NEU.0000370247.11479.B6.

24. Dorresteijn K, Jellema K, van de Beek D, Brouwer MC. Factors and measures predicting external CSF drain-associated ventriculitis: a review and meta-analysis. *Neurology.* 2019;93(22):964-972. doi:10.1212/WNL.0000000000008552.

25. Tunkel AR, Hasbun R, Bhimraj A, et al. 2017 Infectious Diseases Society of America's clinical practice guidelines for healthcare-associated ventriculitis and meningitis. *Clin Infect Dis.* 2017;64(6):e34-e65. doi:10.1093/cid/ciw861.

26. Remeš F, Tomáš R, Jindrák V, Vaniš V, Setlik M. Intraventricular and lumbar intrathecal administration of antibiotics in postneurosurgical patients with meningitis and/or ventriculitis in a serious clinical state. *J Neurosurg.* 2013;119(6):1596-1602. doi:10.3171 /2013.6.JNS122126.

27. Shofty B, Neuberger A, Naffaa ME, et al. Intrathecal or intraventricular therapy for post-neurosurgical gram-negative meningitis: matched cohort study. *Clin Microbiol Infect.* 2016;22(1):66-70. doi:10.1016/j.cmi.2015.09.023.

28. Cina CS, Abouzahr L, Arena GO, Lagana A, Devereaux PJ, Farrokhyar F. Cerebrospinal fluid drainage to prevent paraplegia during thoracic and thoracoabdominal aortic aneurysm surgery: a systematic review and meta-analysis. *J Vasc Surg.* 2004;40(1):36-44. doi:10.1016/j.jvs.2004.03.017.

29. Wynn MM, Mell MW, Tefera G, Hoch JR, Acher CW. Complications of spinal fluid drainage in thoracoabdominal aortic aneurysm repair: a report of 486 patients treated from 1987 to 2008. *J Vasc Surg.* 2009;49(1):29-34; discussion 34-35. doi:10.1016/j. jvs.2008.07.076.

30. Alqaim M, Cosar E, Crawford AS, et al. Lumbar drain complications in patients undergoing fenestrated or branched endovascular aortic aneurysm repair: development of an institutional protocol for lumbar drain management. *J Vasc Surg.* 2020;72(5):1576-1583. doi:10.1016/j.jvs.2020.02.013.

31. Plotkin A, Han SM, Weaver FA, et al. Complications associated with lumbar drain placement for endovascular aortic repair. *J Vasc Surg.* 2021;73(5):1513-1524 e2. doi:10.1016/j.jvs.2020.08.150.

32. Motoyama Y, Nakajima T, Takamura Y, et al. Risk of brain herniation after craniotomy with lumbar spinal drainage: a propensity score analysis. *J Neurosurg.* 2018:1-11. doi:10.3171/2017.12.JNS172215.

33. Lane BC, Scranton R, Cohen-Gadol AA. Risk of brain herniation after craniotomy with preoperative lumbar spinal drainage: a single-surgeon experience of 365 patients among 3000 major cranial cases. *Oper Neurosurg (Hagerstown).* 2021;20(2):E77-E82. doi:10.1093/ons/opaa262.

34. Wang K, Liu Z, Chen X, Lou M, Yin J. Clinical characteristics and outcomes of patients with cerebral herniation during continuous lumbar drainage. *Turk Neurosurg.* 2013;23(5):653-657. doi:10.5137/1019-5149.JTN.7954-13.0.

35. Murad A, Ghostine S, Colohan AR. Controlled lumbar drainage in medically refractory increased intracranial pressure: a safe and effective treatment. *Acta Neurochir Suppl.* 2008;102:89-91. doi:10.1007/978-3-211-85578-2_18.

36. Nasi D, Dobran M, Iacoangeli M, Di Somma L, Gladi M, Scerrati M. Paradoxical brain herniation after decompressive craniectomy provoked by drainage of subdural hygroma. *World Neurosurg.* 2016;91:673 e1-e4. doi:10.1016/j.wneu.2016.04.041.

37. Bhatjiwale MM, Bhatjiwale MG, Chandorkar SS. Transtentorial brain herniation after lumbar drainage in patient planned for cranioplastic reconstruction: catastrophic play between atmospheric and intracranial pressure. *World Neurosurg.* 2019;127:366-369. doi:10.1016/j.wneu.2019.04.090.

38. Zhao J, Li G, Zhang Y, Zhu X, Hou K. Sinking skin flap syndrome and paradoxical herniation secondary to lumbar drainage. *Clin Neurol Neurosurg.* 2015;133:6-10. doi:10.1016/j.clineuro.2015.03.010.

39. Leffert L, Butwick A, Carvalho B, et al. The Society for Obstetric Anesthesia and Perinatology Consensus Statement on the anesthetic management of pregnant and postpartum women receiving thromboprophylaxis or higher dose anticoagulants. *Anesth Analg.* 2018;126(3):928-944. doi:10.1213/ANE.0000000000002530.

40. Horlocker TT, Vandermeuelen E, Kopp SL, Gogarten W, Leffert LR, Benzon HT. Regional anesthesia in the patient receiving antithrombotic or thrombolytic therapy: American Society of Regional Anesthesia and Pain Medicine Evidence-Based Guidelines (Fourth Edition). *Reg Anesth Pain Med.* 2018;43(3):263-309. doi:10.1097/AAP.0000000000000763.

41. Al-Mutair A, Bednar DA. Spinal epidural hematoma. *J Am Acad Orthop Surg.* 2010;18(8):494-502. doi:10.5435/00124635-201008000-00006.

42. Anno M, Yamazaki T, Hara N, Ito Y. The incidence, clinical features, and a comparison between early and delayed onset of postoperative spinal epidural hematoma. *Spine (Phila Pa 1976).* 2019;44(6):420-423. doi:10.1097/BRS.0000000000002838.

43. Leverstein-van Hall MA, Hopmans TE, van der Sprenkel JW, et al. A bundle approach to reduce the incidence of external ventricular and lumbar drain-related infections. *J Neurosurg.* 2010;112(2):345-353. doi:10.3171/2009.6.JNS09223.

44. Schade RP, Schinkel J, Visser LG, Van Dijk JM, Voormolen JH, Kuijper EJ. Bacterial meningitis caused by the use of ventricular or lumbar cerebrospinal fluid catheters. *J Neurosurg.* 2005;102(2):229-234. doi:10.3171/jns.2005.102.2.0229.

45. Citerio G, Signorini L, Bronco A, et al. External ventricular and lumbar drain device infections in ICU patients: a prospective multicenter Italian study. *Crit Care Med.* 2015;43(8):1630-1637. doi:10.1097/CCM.0000000000001019.

46. Coplin WM, Avellino AM, Kim DK, Winn HR, Grady MS. Bacterial meningitis associated with lumbar drains: a retrospective cohort study. *J Neurol Neurosurg Psychiatry.* 1999;67(4):468-473. doi:10.1136/jnnp.67.4.468.